THE TALE OF A WIDOW'S ANGUISH

THE TALE OF A WIDOW'S ANGUISH

Haiwata Manrou

ATHENA PRESS
LONDON

THE TALE OF A WIDOW'S ANGUISH
Copyright © Haiwata Manrou 2006

All Rights Reserved

No part of this book may be reproduced in any form
by photocopying or by any electronic or mechanical means,
including information storage and retrieval systems,
without permission in writing from both the copyright
owner and the publisher of this book.

ISBN 1 84401 618 8

First Published 2006 by
ATHENA PRESS
Queen's House, 2 Holly Road
Twickenham TW1 4EG
United Kingdom

Printed for Athena Press

Sincere thanks to all the readers.

I was born in a small village seventy years ago in the country of Guyana, former British Guiana, where the British ruled. The official language was English but Hindi and Arabic were spoken by some of the older people. The small village I lived in was called Hague, on the west coast of Demerara.

★

The first tragic event in my life occurred when I was two years old – my mother died during childbirth, leaving alive a healthy baby boy. He was adopted by one of my aunts who had no children of her own. This aunt was a great character, big and bossy. I was left with my father as he figured out how to cope with us.

I had an elder sister, who at that time, was five years old. We had several farms and Dad was very busy. The neighbours promised to help and some elderly relatives became our nannies. Everyone in the village was called uncle or auntie – it was like an extended family.

Our house was fairly large, with frontage and about half an acre of back garden that was lined with tropical fruits for every season and tall and stately coconut trees. A large pond was in the corner of the land and connected to it was a small trench so the pond could fill up with sweet, black water from a nearby creek.

We had a dog, lots of chickens and laying hens. Dad used the eggs for baking and cooking. We also had cows, for milk was essential for our daily use and for making homemade butter. The mature coconut was used for delicious drinks and ice cubes were used to cool it. The dry coconut was grated and made into oil for home use. We performed this process once a month so that there was always a supply.

From the age of five, I attended school some three to four miles away. I had to walk to and from, as there was no bus service at that time. Sometimes a school teacher would give you a lift on their bicycle bar. This was a real treat as the sun was very hot and the dusty roads made you tired. I really enjoyed my schooldays. Unfortunately, I had to leave at eleven years old. This was a very sad day in my life; I wanted, so badly, to get some sort of qualification so that I could pursue a career in nursing.

Village life was good, although our neighbours had many babies who died before the age of three. Tuberculosis was rampant, as were polio and malaria. Men from the Environmental Health department used to spray the drains with DDT to keep the mosquitoes at bay; over our beds were net curtains. One of my best friends died of malaria. That was a devastating time for me. She was only twelve years old. There was some treatment available, but the district doctor was eight miles away and he only visited when someone was dying. Desperate for an answer, I asked myself how this could happen. I began asking more questions: what went wrong? Why was the doctor not notified? Why was she not taken to the public hospital? However, the hospital was nine miles away and you had to cross over to the town by ferryboat to get there.

Transportation was very poor indeed. It took all day to get from place to place. Most people walked or rode bicycles. There was a bus service and a railway but these were by no means regular.

After leaving school I spent most of my time helping some neighbours, who were seamstresses, to add some finishing touches to their garments. I would pick their brains whilst helping out so that I also gained some knowledge.

*

My family background was good. My father – we called him Daddy – was a farmer and had really green fingers; everything he planted gave him a good return. My sister and I had to water the plants twice daily, before we went to school and late afternoons. We enjoyed each other's company. Because Daddy was on the farm all day we spent a lot of time together whilst we were growing up. Dad employed a lady to come in each day to teach us how to cook, wash, iron our clothing and other household chores.

*

A difficult time ahead was signalled when neighbours began gossiping that we were about to have a mother and that our dad had several lady friends, but only one would be the lucky lady. My sister and I were asked to go to stay with our aunt – my dad's sister – who lived in the next

The Tale of a Widow's Anguish

county, on the west coast of Demerara. During that time we saw all the other family members, including Dad's seven brothers and his old, grumpy sister. She was very mean and liked to work us from morning to night.

We packed and went to Aunt Nora, no hugs or kisses to welcome us. That is what I missed – starved of maternal love. Orders were given by Aunt Nora that we were not to ride the bicycle that her son owned. No climbing trees, either, as this was a boy's hobby. She was so miserable at times, I used to cry most nights. She made us sleep on the floor – no mattress, just some old sheets thrown on the floor. I wanted so much to run away, as I was so unhappy and missed my home with Dad. I thought I would be better off dead. I did not manage to confide in anyone; my mind was running riot within me.

During this time, a message came to say my dad was coming at the weekend. There would be a party with all the family. I was curious about what was going on. Then the big bombshell was dropped. Gossip again, from one of the family members, said my dad was going to be married in a few weeks and that the lady did not like children, so we would have to move in with our aunt.

Forsaken, I thought, in desperation, I would have to end my life; I had to make a plan. Searching for ways, I came across some rat poison in an old shed. I took some and held it in my hands and went to a nearby riverbank, where I sat and drank it, then plunged in. I was carried along for a little while, then found myself trapped in some heavy moss near the bank. I was coughing for a long time, then came up, sat on the bank and cried my eyes out. I went back to face reality.

★

The weekend arrived. Dad came, the family gathered, some ate and drank too much; Aunty called me a tomboy as I was obsessed with fishing and climbing. I overheard that my sister was to stay at my aunt's after Dad got married but I would be staying with Dad. In the background there was lots of noise and big quarrels going on about why we would be separated. After the weekend, Dad, my sister and myself went home together.

*

In the third week of being back home, Dad got married with a large gathering of neighbours and nearly the whole village invited to the wedding. I wondered what my new mother would be like to live with.

I viewed her physical appearance. She was tall and slim with long dark hair. Strangely, all her teeth were gold. She had an hilarious laugh and all the gold would shine; I took a dislike to her, based on her laugh. The lady next door had a lodger called Igal, and he told us some fairy stories, saying if someone had gold teeth, they must not tell lies because if they did, all their teeth would fall out. My stepmother's teeth never fell out, even though she told many lies.

She made up stories about my sister and I. When we challenged her she became angry – she was very hot-tempered and loudmouthed, and she called us names that I am ashamed to repeat. Hell was let loose one day, with a good beating from her because we told her to go back to where she came from. My dad was so much in love with her that he had little to say to her about it. Many evenings we were starved; Dad would give us some of the food from his plate. I did not mind too much but my sister loved her food. I would pick some fruits and eat them and drink plenty of milk to keep me going. However, it became unbearable and my dear sister left home and went to live with my dad's sister – the bossy one.

I was devastated and angry at the whole situation and thought about running away. I had an aunt – my mother's sister – who lived some five miles away, so I thought I would go to her house and ask if she could put me up for a while until I found a job or something to do. Off I went, and was accepted by my aunt's mother-in-law. She said I could stay but must help with the cooking and washing. I said yes to everything, but at that time, aged thirteen, I could only cook simple food and only cook for a few people.

Feeling insecure and incapable of carrying out my part of the deal, I was unable to sleep. I spoke to my aunt, as we shared the same room. I asked her how many people were living in the house and how much food was to be prepared. She gave a great sigh and began to cry. I too start crying, sobbing very loudly. In the next room I heard a loud voice saying, 'I will shoot you dead, Sarah!' That was my aunt's husband. I was petrified, frightened out of my mind. Aunt Sarah whispered to me to be quiet, saying he would do it – that's the sort of a person he was.

I was told that there were twelve people living in the house and that food had to be prepared for all. Out of those, two were Sarah's children – a boy and a girl. She was about four years old, very pretty and had olive skin like her mum.

The next day I could not face the challenge and resolved to go with my aunt to help with cutting grass to feed the cows. This was her job, but she also had to cook and wash for all the family. Her mother-in-law did nothing, only swept the house and gossiped about the family.

I was curious about the situation and began to ask some questions. Aunt Sarah said the man she married had been her secret lover and that she had run away from her family. She went on to say that in those days, marriage had to be arranged and, because her lover was a Hindu and she was a Christian, they were not suitable for marriage. Unfortunately, my grandparents had both died when Mum and Sarah were children, and they were adopted by their godparents, who had lived with them in their parents' home, before they had died. The property was left to the two sisters. Then, mum got married and Aunt Sarah left home.

Aunt Sarah began saying that when she gave birth to the little girl, her husband said it was not his child, because she was too fair skinned, especially considering his son was very dark, like himself. She said that he had hated her from that day on and had not spoken to her for ten years. I decided to go back home to my dad, visiting my aunt once a month to talk about our maltreatment at home. There was no way for either of us to escape from this dreadful life.

*

Eventually Aunt Sarah died at the age of thirty-two – from mental torture. This was a very sad day for me. I lost a lot of weight, as I was unable to eat or sleep; this was the only person who I could confide in. All hope had gone. I would have to find someone else who would listen to me. There was a neighbour who seemed very kind. We used to meet up at the well where we drew water for cooking and washing. I called him Uncle Igal.

The Tale of a Widow's Anguish

He would ask how I was being treated and I would say, 'the Tiger' – meaning my stepmother – 'does not like me and I do not like her.' He said I must try and abide and one day I would be able to get married and leave home. That thought gave me some hope.

The persecution went on, even when the Tiger was expecting a baby. I hoped with all my heart it would be a girl. I had false hope as it turned out to be a boy, and I took a dislike to him. As my mother had died after having a baby boy, dad was pleased and I became the housemaid. When the child cried she would scream at me to go and rock him in a hammock. Probably he had wind, thinking back. Eventually, however, I got to like the little chap. I thought she would become kind and share her love with me. At times she would hug and kiss him. I used to get jealous wishing for someone to give me a hug.

One day, a message arrived to say that I should visit the aunt with whom my sister was staying. I had mixed feelings, as I was unsure as to why I had to go, but I thought it would make a change for me to get away from that beastly woman for a week or two. Dad took me at the weekend and all the family gathered as my sister was to be engaged – this was an arranged marriage. My sister had a year of courtship with her husband-to-be. She spoke nicely about him, but she wanted to get married in the church. His father would not give consent for his son to be married in a church as they were Hindus. I was glad for her but sad that she could not have a church wedding. Dad did not mind, as my aunt and uncle were in control of the situation.

My sister and I spoke of the wedding and how it might be possible for me to go and live with her after she had settled in her new home.

The weekend ended and I had to return home to help the Tiger and her baby. I began to wish it was I who was going to be married, but I really didn't want marriage; I wanted a career. But how could I achieve this without further education? I would have loved to go back to school or get some private tuition on the basics – maths and English. I had to pluck up the courage to ask Dad if he would pay for me to have some private tuition. I met up with him while he was milking the cows and told him what I would like to do. He promised to make some enquiries as to where I could go. However, news got out and the Tiger, my stepmother, started a big quarrel with my dad, saying it would be a waste of money and it was about time I was married and left home.

This was the time to retaliate – I refused to help to look after my step-brother, now that she was helping on the farm and keeping an eye on Dad to make sure he did not go to town to look into getting me some private schooling. I thought she must have been psychic because that was a secret between dad and myself. However, she was expecting another baby and this time it was a girl. I hoped things would get better for me, but they only got worse.

One day she found in my room a song I'd written down: 'Oh my darling, Oh my darling, Clementine'. Well, she exploded saying that I had a boyfriend and that this was a letter she had found in my room. She told the whole neighbourhood, as well as Igal, who was my friend. He told her it was a song that I'd heard on the radio. It was true. I would go across to our neighbour's place and sit on his bridge, listening to his radio with a pen and paper to write anything down that I thought would be worth knowing. It gave me a few hours of peace and quiet, listening to something good. That was a small amount of joy I had for myself and it was taken away from me. Now, Tigress came over to me with the supposed letter in her hand. I managed to snatch it off her and tore it. She exploded – her arm extended and she got hold of my long hair, swinging me from side to side. Then she picked up a coconut broom and beat me with it. I began to shout for help. My dress was torn, my whole body was striped with bruises. I was shaking with fear but managed to break loose and went to see a neighbour. I thought she was going to kill me.

The neighbour started shouting at her, saying our mother would be crying in her grave to see the cruelty inflicted on her daughter. Dad came home. She told him about this piece of paper but was unable to show anything of it because it had been torn to shreds. However, Uncle Igar came over and told Dad that it was a song and not a letter, that I had been chastised for nothing, and Dad should do something about it, otherwise, he would take me to the police station and report the matter. It appears Dad cautioned her but she would not accept it.

Later that week there was lots going on, as Tigress packed and left Dad with her two children. I went home and after a week Dad said that if I wanted to go and live with my aunt, he would make some arrangements with her, because my sister was getting married in a few weeks' time and they would be glad of some help.

Dad visited my stepmother, who said that unless I left the house she would not return. I packed and went to live with my aunt. However, the Tigress came home unwell so she needed my help. Dad came to fetch me but I refused to go. I told my sister and auntie I would rather die than go back home.

★

Wedding bells rang. My sister got married. All went well and she looked like a fairy on the day. She went and set up home with her husband. They were a happy couple. They always invited me to stay as long as I wanted. I was a sensitive person and liked staying with my aunt, although she worked me hard. I did not mind because, at last, there were no more beatings. My uncle was nice and he would chat to me and I could ask him questions about the war that was going on in Britain, I was interested because some of my cousins were recruited and joined the RAF. I kept in contact with one of them until he was shot and killed in Cyprus in the mid-Fifties.

Late afternoons, when everyone was at home, I used to sit with my uncle and he would ask me to recite the times-tables, one to twelve, and also to read the clock with its roman numbers. It was an educational few hours that I cherished. In return, I used to mend his trousers – often the knees would get torn and my lazy aunt was not good with needle and cotton, so I had this little job. He would give me some money to buy sweets, which I was grateful for. My dad would send money for my keep and some pocket money, which I saved up each week in the hope that I would find someone to give me some private tuition.

Time went on and it seemed less and less likely that I would be able to find a career. Now, my sister was expecting her first baby and she was preparing for the big day; in those days, all babies were born at home. A midwife was booked. She lived in the village and got on her bicycle when she was called out to her patient.

My sister gave birth to a bouncing baby girl. She did

not cry much, she was very peaceful indeed. I loved her to bits; until this day she is my favourite niece. She is now married and working and living in Jamaica.

*

In those days, my brother-in-law was working away from home and it was company for my sister to have me staying with her. I went to see my aunt and uncle regularly, as they were good to me. I made some friends, including the girl next door, who was my age. She was attending high school in the town. Her father was very wealthy and owned many houses and much land. Her parents were kind and loved to share their time and money. Her name was Yvonne and she would give me her books to read. We used to talk about what we were going to do when we were older. I was hell bent on becoming a nurse. My friend said she would like to get married. I really liked my friend's mother; she made me feel wanted and cared for. It was the tenderness and love I so craved. At last I felt happy.

I thought the evil that persecuted my soul was gone. I could safely confide in my friend's mum, tell her the things that troubled me. Her voice made me feel secure. I rejoiced. My sister was also a great help in reassuring me that life would get better one day. Cast down, but not forsaken. I was grateful for this time in my life. How long it would last, I didn't know.

My brother-in-law returned home to find his new baby. He was overjoyed, and thanked me for my kind help in looking after my sister and his home during his absence. He had a few weeks' leave and I enjoyed being there as well. He was extremely kind to me and often sat and chatted with me, asking what I wanted to do with my life; he was like a big brother to me.

This is why I found it difficult to understand what happened next. One night as I was sleeping in a room next to my sister's, I felt a strong weight over my body. I thought it was a dream, but it was a real encounter. My brother-in-law was over me and started to kiss and hug me. I pushed him away and asked him what he was doing, and told him that it was not right. I managed to light a lamp, as in those days, there was no electricity in the village. Well, this was the last straw. I so much wanted to scream and shout for my sister. But I thought that he would throw me out and, as it was night, I wouldn't be able to wake my friend's mother. So I stayed awake for the rest of the night. It was the longest night of my life. I cry my eyes out thinking about it.

The next morning, I had no breakfast, but visited the neighbour and asked her if I could have a word with her. She made me a drink and I started crying, telling her of my episode with my brother-in-law. She was disgusted and went to see my sister to tell her what had happened.

Well, she was sad for me and asked what I wanted to do. But I was to promise not to tell my father. I went berserk asking how could all this evil befall me.

A message was sent to my dad saying I would return home to live with them. Very disheartened, I went back home and a few days later we visited a distant uncle who promised to take me in. He was a farmer and had lots of paddy fields. He hired labourers to thrash and cut the paddy in the fields. Things were done manually in those days. I asked my uncle if I could go in the field to cut the paddy and he agreed, but said it was hard work and the stalks would bruise my little arms. I told him to give me a

The Tale of a Widow's Anguish

try. Well, he gave me a few rods that I had to cut and put into bundles so the men could take them and the bullock and cart could deliver them to the barn. I made good progress but also made some clumsy bundles. No one bothered too much as long as the paddy was cut and put in the barn before the rain came.

I was tired but delighted with what I had accomplished in the week. I was paid forty dollars, which I thought was great. I was at last getting somewhere. It was sad that I couldn't see my sister and my sweet niece I was so fond of, but I thought I should try to forget the saga. I was deeply hurt inside and unable to trust anyone anymore.

★

Time went by, and I met a hawker's daughter who became friendly with me. She would help to collect money for her mother at weekends. Sometimes she asked questions about why I was not living at my own home. I confided in her and also spoke of my desire to become a nurse, She was educated and said that her mother might be able to help me pursue a career. My uncle was kind and helpful, but said it would be nice for me to get married and settle down, since I was eighteen years old, coming on nineteen. A few months later my friend said her mother and my uncle had arranged to call and see my father about me getting married to one of her cousins. I said no, but she said that they were rich and I would have a chance to study and educate myself because they were living in town. I told her I did not approve because, now I was earning money, I would be able to pay for private tuition.

★

All was arranged and many months went by before I was to be married to some strange person I had never met and didn't know anything about. I had to agree because it was the custom that all girls got married before they reached twenty. The wedding took place in the town. Some family came and a Hindu ceremony was performed in the late afternoon. Seeing this man for the first time he looked much older than I thought he'd be. He seemed pleasant, even though we did not speak – we were not allowed to at this point in time. I went through the whole ordeal speechless; I did not understand anything that was going on. No one explained to me what was going to happen. I was so desperately unhappy.

To my knowledge, it was not a legal marriage, although I was dressed up like a bride, all in white. Afterwards, I went out for a ride with this strange man who was my husband and his brother. After the drive, they took some photographs of my so-called husband and myself. Later we met up with our parents, who looked very pleased with themselves.

Everyone went home and I was to be an obedient slave for the rest of my life. Now I had to think hard. I had exchanged one chain for another. I was nineteen now and everyone expected me to be a good housewife and have lots of children.

The mother-in-law was a tyrant and I was not to behave in an unruly fashion or else she would tell her son who would give me a hiding. There was not much love or romance; he was a very cold man. He came home from work, ate and slept and demanded sex. Oh, how I hated the mess I was in but I was unable to do anything.

The Tale of a Widow's Anguish

His mother was very aggressive and she knew how to throw bullets for her son to fire at me; she would tell him stories about where I went and what I did. Late evenings, I would go out feeling like a big empty ship, being tossed about, with nowhere to dock. That year, I became a mother and gave birth to a baby girl.

We had to live in one small room; in it was an area where I had to cook for five people: his mother, father grandmother, my husband and myself. My life was another hell. I found the courage to visit my sister and did not say anything of the past. I buried it in my heart. I told my sister that my husband was married already. I had found a photograph of him and his wife, but I was afraid to challenge him.

She thought it would be wise not to say anything, and that I should make plans to leave him and she would stand by me whatever happened. Eighteen months later, I gave birth to a baby boy. He was called Jo. His father seemed to pay some attention to him, because he was a boy, and his grandparents would play with him, but my little girl was not liked, although the great-grandma did sometimes take her out for walks. During the days, I would go out for walks with my little boy and walk into any church I found and pray, asking God to help me get out of this helpless situation. One day I met up with a churchgoer. I felt I could talk to her. I began to tell her that I had come to expect the worst in life. I told her that if things ever changed, I would be delighted.

This lady seemed to want to listen and showed empathy with my situation. She told me that I should speak nicely to my common-law husband and ask him to go to the ministry and put our names down to re-housed because the Government had set up a scheme for people with young children who had bad accommodation and were over-crowded. I felt good and finally thought that God did care.

That evening, I mustered the courage to speak to John – that was his name – and I told him that I understood we could get a nice house from the Government, but we would need a down payment of $100. He agreed but said he had no money. I told him of my savings in the Post Office, and that I would pay the deposit. A few weeks went by. He did not go to sign up for the house. I began to despair. I thought I would write to the governor. Pen to paper, I wrote a letter to Governor Savage at Government House, asking him to look into my situation and if only it were so, as I had two small children and was living in a kitchen.

*

Showers of blessings! Two weeks later, a lady from the Housing Department came to visit me. She asked my mother-in-law, who had a shop in the front of the house, to see me and the children. She was refused. The lady told her it was urgent and that the request came from Government officials. It was raining that day and there was water leaking near the bed and by the side of the cradle I had placed a bucket to catch the drips. The lady came in but there was nowhere for her to sit. She asked me how I was coping and I broke down in tears. She gripped my shoulder firmly, saying I shouldn't worry, as I would be re-housed soon. A few months later, we heard from the Housing Department stating we would be given a two-bedroom house in the scheme and we were given the location. I was delighted.

The Tale of a Widow's Anguish

The down-payment was to be paid quickly and then monthly instalments for the next ten years. Because the country was run by the British, things were done quickly.

My mother-in-law did not take kindly to this. Only John's name was to be on the contract, since we were not legally married. I did not mind; I would be able to work and save some more money.

*

Moving time. We had no furniture – nothing except one bed – and my little girl, Babs, would have to sleep with us until we could buy her one of her own. Jo's cradle was put into the next room. We had some nice people move in next door, with three children. They were to be a tower of strength for me. The lady was called Olga and her husband, who was an electrician, worked in town. We called him Uncle Norman.

At weekends they would invite me and the children over for meals with their families. I still hated John but accepted the situation for the time being; life was more bearable, and I had my hands full with the two children. My neighbour had her elderly father living with her and he was so sweet and kind to me. He often helped me with the children, while I went out to buy food. He played a great role as a granddad to them and I loved him very much. This was a person who I could trust and I told him all my troubles. He often said that life would get better after the kids had grown up.

*

Well, I had to get a job. I would try to get a sewing machine on HP from the Singer company. Olga suggested that I pay a down-payment and then borrow the rest of the money from my dad or sister and pay them back when I started the sewing business. I got the money to pay for the machine and told all the neighbours to spread the news that I would sew clothing for a small charge. I was no seamstress but had some knowledge of how to put clothing together. I was eager and full of confidence that I could make a go of it. John made no progress – he was the same cold man who was not interested in me. He sat every evening, sleeping in the rocking chair; he would only contribute a little money, so now I was paying all the bills. My sewing became established through word of mouth. How I was able to make all those stylish dresses, only God knows. I cut paper patterns using newspaper from the neighbours. I would visit the town to look at the clothing in the shop windows and start drawing the various patterns. That is how I did it. I even made a pattern for wedding dresses. Then I began baking and icing cakes. This too took off and I was well on my way, although John's mother would still pay nosy visits and make rude comments (which I ignored). Neighbours helped me with looking after the children. I sewed for their families and themselves for free because they were so kind to me.

*

One day I was told that the stores in town were looking for a seamstress to make all kinds of garments for their store, and they would provide all the material and pay for each piece of work. Well, I had to be bold and get the job. I undid some of my children's clothing, the nice pieces that were given to them, and, following their pattern, made some new ones as a sample.

I took them with me to the shop and asked if I could see the person in charge about the advert. A smart, stocky chap came out and spoke to me. He asked if I'd ever done bulk work before. I said no, but if he were to give me a trial, I would be very grateful. I showed him my sample and he was rather pleased. He said I was clever and he would supply all the materials needed that very day. The orders were given and they ran into hundreds of baby dresses and jumpsuits for me to make. I was very nervous, but did not show it; I had it in my head that success only came once, and I must grab it with both hands.

I had to get a taxi to take me home. I shared my joy with Olga and her dad. He reassured me of his help at all times, which I was grateful for. I had a deadline for when I had to finish sewing all these garments. I used to work till two in the morning. I was so tired and exhausted, but was determined to get on. I just had to fill in the stock and I would have a month of rest, which I would use to take the children to see Dad and my sister. John was not interested, so I would go away for weekends but I had to get back to cook and wash and tidy-up; men never cooked in those days or helped in the house.

With time to seek further education, I went to join the British Red Cross, as well as the Young Women's Christian Association. I enrolled in the home-nursing course with the Red Cross, as well as attending meetings at the YWCA. I met lots of important people from abroad. It was educational; I would only listen at the time, not saying too much because I was not educated and had little knowledge, but afterwards I would ask questions about the subject-matter. They were all very kind and I was well treated. One lady in particular, who was a retired headmistress called Miss Wilson, took an interest in me. I told her of my plans but was ashamed to let her know that I was not educated. All night, the thought haunted me but I saw that this was an opportunity for me to get help, so I must put away pride. Out goes my pride. At the next meeting I spoke to Miss Wilson about giving me some private tuition and I told her that I would be willing to pay for it, whatever the cost. My luck was in; she welcomed the idea.

Now I was about to broaden my horizons. My sewing business was still going on and I had lots of homework to do. I passed home-nursing with flying colours and went on to do a first-aid course, along with my English and maths. With the children and the chores, I had little time to sleep. It was tiring but rewarding, and I was on the way to accomplishing some of what I wanted to do.

Bills were paid, money was in the bank, and Miss Wilson gave me lessons free, for which I am for ever grateful. Indeed, I am grateful to all the people whom I met, and especially for the never-ending help from my good neighbours.

Time was moving on and the two children were going to school, not far from home. They were well behaved and adjusted to us living away from Grandma, whom they would visit after school. I would play with them and play some hide-and-seek with the other children in the neighbourhood. They would laugh and giggle; how I loved to see them happy. I gave them lots of hugs and kisses, something that I never had.

*

The Tale of a Widow's Anguish

Fortunes changed. Four years had passed and I was pregnant for the third time. I was frantic. My whole world had collapsed; this was the last thing I wanted. I was very depressed, unable to do anything about the situation. However, I continued to carry on as normal. Luckily I had no pregnancy ailments – I was tough as an old boot.

I continued to work late into the night. I was cross with John. When I told my sister, she said I must have the baby in a private hospital and then be sterilised so as not to have any more babies. I gave birth at home with the help of kind Olga and her father.

I hired a nanny who looked after little Tom. I did breastfeed him, as I had with the other two, as it was the done thing in those days. I went to a private hospital and asked if I could have my tubes done. They refused as I was too young and consent had to be given by John. I was furious; I would not have him demanding sex any more.

Months went by and I became very unhappy. I was unable to sleep or eat; I was not putting on weight. Discussing the situation with Olga, she said I had to give up some of my activities. By then I had gained a first-aid certificate and was well able to do some maths and write basic letters. My mental capacity was well stretched; I was heading for a breakdown.

One late afternoon, I felt I was walking in the air while cooking. I rushed over to Olga. She was awfully sweet. She told John that I was to see a doctor immediately. He shrugged, saying I was OK. Olga was furious, and she and her husband took me to see a doctor in Georgetown. It cost quite a bit but Olga paid the fee. He said I had post-natal depression, made worse by stress and work and advised me to take a break from home. Well, this was not good news. My dad and sister came to see if they could help. The children went to stay with my sister. The store manager was kind, saying I could have a break as they had a good stock of the things I made. A holiday was booked for two weeks in the West Indies, which I paid for. It cost $99.

I went and met up with some nice people, and taking Valium – 2 mg – and not having to work, or do anything, I began to feel better. But soon the holiday ended and I had to return home and begin to pick up the pieces. While I was on holiday, there had been a fire in the town and the stores I worked for were burnt down. This was shattering news for me and I did not know what I would do. However, the manager reassured me by saying I would be able to get some work as and when the shop was refurbished. I was still able to do some sewing for the people living nearby and this kept me going. I still had some money in the bank but I would not spend any more as this was my get-away money and I had to keep it – my very own secret.

I was better and continued my private tuition and doing meals-on-wheels while Granddad looked after Tom. He was a happy chap.

There was not much work from the store but I did not mind as I was having more time with the children and that was a first for me. The days were nice and we all went picnicking once a week.

*

New lover for John, so the saying goes. I did not mind at all; I was glad for someone to take him over as I did not find any love or romance in him. He was just too old for me and I still had my secret plan to run away. I told my sister and asked if she would look after the children for me while I worked for three years, training. She agreed. But how? My thinking cap on, I went to see the Matron at the local hospital. She was kind but to the point. She said I would have to pass an entrance test in maths and English. I told her I would try, given a chance. We discussed my education and she continued, saying that the waiting list for training was three years and it would be better if I applied for training in the UK, as they were recruiting. Having said that, she told me if I failed the test then I could work as a nursing aid because I had some training from the Red Cross. This would come in handy and I could try again to further my education. Encouraging news, I thought.

I made further enquiries into the training in the UK. I had a British passport and money in the bank; I only needed to get John to agree for me to leave the children. Very tricky matter. By this time he had many women and did not care what happened to me. I too was glad of this situation. Well, I put on my charm and asked him if I could go study for nursing. Oh, he said, you have a new man who is putting you up to all sorts of things. I took a few slaps because I back-chatted him but I told him no matter what happened, I would become a nurse.

Nothing more was said for the time being. I signed papers, they asked for references, and I found a ship which was sailing in January for the port of Southampton. The children were on my mind; how could I work out what to do? I spoke to Olga, pondering all this.

Now, could I be so daring as to put a career before my children? This was hellish. My head was turning, accusing myself of being selfish, and wondering what I would tell the children. I told myself I was good in a crisis, but not this time; sleepless nights. I went to stay with my sister, as it was holiday time for the children and talked things over with her. Leaving the children, for three years would be tough but I would visit when I got my holiday. We talked and she was very clear about my plans; she volunteered to look after the three children, if John would allow her to keep them. My sister said she would go to see his mother because, after all, I was not married to John and was free to leave the country. Now I had my spokesperson, I felt good, and would take up the offer; whatever happened I had dreams I had to fulfil.

*

I had made up my mind, and my ticket was booked to the UK. Drastic action now, I managed to tell John some story that I was going on a holiday and the children would be taken care of by my sister – did he approve? He made a lot of fuss, very threatening behaviour, saying I would never leave the country in one piece. I was disciplined by his mother, who said if I tried to run away I would be killed. Well, I froze, and did not utter a word for a few hours until he left the house. I took the children and went to see my kind neighbour and told her what the situation was.

She told me that I must be very careful. John did not come home for many days. I was pleased – I had two weeks to pack and leave my home. I bought a suitcase and left it with Olga; all packing of my clothing was done by her. She was a tower of strength for me. I tried to coach the children as far as possible and told them I would be back soon, that I was going job-hunting further afield.

My sister went to see John's mother and told her that I would be away from the country for a while to collect my thoughts. It appears she did not say much in reply. Two days later, I went to my sister's house with the children and my few things along with my suitcase. John did not follow me – so far, so good.

We hired a taxi to take me to the airport. Only my sister and a family friend knew of my plans. I flew from Timery airport to Trinidad, where I stayed overnight in a hotel. My heart was sad, telling me that I had made a mistake. The farewell was anguish indeed. I cried so much on the plane that the airhostess thought I was going to a funeral. However, the clock could not be turned back.

*

Settled into the hotel for the night but unable to sleep, I read through all the travelling documents and about the hospital where I was going. Next day, I ate very little and set out to join the Spanish boat.

I boarded the ship and was shown to the cabin I would share with one other person who was going to the UK. At least we had something in common, but I still resolved not to give away too much about myself; I was travelling under my maiden name. The ship would reach Britain in twenty-eight days – a long time to be sailing. During our journey, the ship docked at ten ports. We were allowed to go out and spend few hours at each, which helped relieve the monotony. It took away the boredom of the seas.

One morning, as I was ironing a dress, I met up with a Jamaican lady, named Sarah. She seemed amicable and wanted to talk and she asked where I would be staying when I got to the UK. I told her I was going to pursue a career. She was pleased for me and said we should keep in contact. It appeared she was married and had been on holiday but was returning to her home. Each day we met up after meals, and when the ship docked we went out together and visited places.

Most nights I couldn't stop thinking of the children and cried my eyes out. I really had a tormented mind. Lots of times I thought I would return home, but was reassured by my sister – I knew she would take care of the children. Some days I was so distressed, I was unable to eat. How I longed to get off that ship; if I had wings I would have flown like a bird to get home and see my children. I had a few books with me, which I read over and over, as I did not wish to get mixed up with other people who might have asked awkward questions.

*

My new world. I arrived at Southampton. Cleared Customs. I had to make my way to the hospital. I got on a train to Waterloo then the Underground and then a bus to the hospital. I got there early in the morning and was escorted by a porter, who said he would send the House Matron to see me. I had cups of tea while I waited. A very smart middle-aged lady came and asked me lots of questions.

To my surprise, she said I was not on the list until August and that I had to wait until the Matron came on duty to see what she would say. Hours went by; I thought I had got it all wrong. I had; there were only two intakes in a year: one in January and the other in August. I had missed the January school.

Later, I was asked to visit Matron's office. She was kind and polite. She asked what I would do and did I have somewhere to go to? I was full of pride and said yes, knowing I was making a big mistake. However, she said I must give her an address where she could contact me. I had Sarah's name and address, which I gave to her, and left in desperation. As there was a call box, I phoned Sarah and asked if she would be kind enough to see me. She gave directions as how to find her house as it was in the area, just a bus ride away. I arrived at her home and told her that I gave her name and address and said that was my contact address. She was awfully sweet and did not mind, saying I could stay with her until I got a flat and a job. I could hardly sleep; we shared the same bed, as her husband was sleeping in the next room with another man. How odd, I thought. No question I was in trouble myself; I had misunderstood my paperwork and had not read it carefully. I decided to go out and seek lodgings. Sarah told me to look in shop windows for adverts from people with rooms to let. Would I be able to pay for lodgings and feed myself? I received a letter from Matron. She told me there was a vacancy in the sewing room and, if I would like to take the job, I must contact the sewing manager. Without hesitation I rang the lady, who said I should come in for an interview the next week and a time was arranged.

I was very homesick and missed the children badly but had to take heart and keep going. I wrote to my sister of my safe arrival but did not mention what was going on. Sarah said I could stay as long as I liked. Her husband was nice, as were all the others who lived in the house. It appears all the rooms were let to men.

As it was winter, I had to get some warm clothing. I managed to get a second-hand coat, which came in handy as I was so cold.

I went to see the sewing manager and she said she would give me a trial during the week. Pleased with myself, when I got home, Sarah was eager to hear of how I had got on. We chatted and talked about how much she would like me to pay for my board and lodging. £5 per week, she said, which I thought was reasonable. The next day I went for the trial job. It was mainly making button-holes and sewing them on to nurses' uniforms, but also some other sewing jobs which I could handle extremely well. The job was mine on a short contract, as PTS would commence in August. I earned about £3 per week.

I received a letter from Matron saying I must come in to undergo an entrance test. It was a worrying week for me; I had to brush up on some maths and English. The day came and I was in a classroom with about ten others, one an Irish lady who never stopped talking while we were writing, asking how you spell this and that. I told her to be quiet or else we might be expelled. The two hours went by and we were told to stop writing. Then we had an oral test, where we were asked why we would like to become nurses. Most people said 'to get a career'. The only thing that came into my head at that moment was that I wanted to help the sick and suffering. Matron gave me a great smile. I was still very tense and anxious of the outcome, but the others seemed more relaxed. We made small-talk; it seemed that most of us were from abroad. Tea was served and we were told to go home and that we would hear from Matron soon.

I was still working in the sewing room, and in the second week, a letter arrived from Matron saying that I was successful and would commence training on the first of August; this was great news and I was so happy.

Now I had to tell my sister that it would take me longer to finish, as I was six months behind. I began to relax but still had the mental torture of leaving the children. No news from John, but my sister was plagued by his mother. She sent letters to me to say the children were happy but eager to see me back.

*

My dream was coming true through PTS. When it started, I found it hard to concentrate on the theory, and while I was good on the wards and enjoyed every minute, it was hard work keeping my mind on the job. One day I felt very lighted-headed. I sat down and the ward sister said I must see a doctor. When I saw one he told me I must be troubled about something, because he could find nothing wrong with me. He advised me to have a few days off. I thought this would be a setback for me as you were not supposed to go off sick while you were in PTS. Well, I thought, I must pull myself out of the depressive mood. I was studying all hours at night and working during the day, with only one and a half days off each week.

*

Exam time and most of us passed, although some had to retake. The fact that I did well said I was making good progress and I was able to give my sister the latest news. With my four weeks' holiday a year, I decided to get a part-time job somewhere, but it was required to be in a field other than nursing. I went to see Sarah from time to time and we became good friends. She told me there was a job advertised in a shop window for curtain makers, so I went to the shop to see about it. The gentleman said it was piece work and payment was in cash. As I was now living in the hospital, and all meals were provided, I had little to worry about. He was a cheat though and he asked me to make coffee every two hours. When I told him I was not a tea-maker, he said he would inform the Home Office that I was living in Britain. I did not tell him I was employed at the hospital. That was the end of that job but I really needed extra cash to go home the following year.

For the rest of the month, I spent most of my time studying, writing letters and making dresses, as we had a sewing machine in the nurses' quarter. I made several for my daughter and bought a few presents to send home for the children. In my second year I met up with a girl who asked if I would like to become a Christian. We went to her room and prayed that God would forgive my sins and I talked to him, telling him of all my troubles.

This was a new start for me. I began to go to church and attend weekday meetings at what was called the International Christian Fellowship. They were a happy bunch and loved to share whatever they had; we would even borrow one another's coats or cardigans. Some nights, when I studied late and got very hungry but had nothing to eat, I would go peeping under my friends' door to see it they had lights on. Then I would knock and they would open the door and share some crackers with me. I was so grateful, and resolved to return the favour when I could. It was rough; once the dining room was closed there was nowhere to eat as it would cost you too much.

*

Time was passing now and I received a letter saying that John did not want anything to do with the children and it was my responsibility to send money for their keep. How would I manage that? I had some savings and would have to send my sister some money each month, but even so, this would be a setback for me and it meant that I would not be able to go on the holiday to see the children. I talked to God about the problem.

I wrote my sister a letter, enclosing a postal order and telling her I will repay her in the future, but in the meantime I would send what I could afford. I had to stop sending presents and get my priorities right.

I never told anyone of my past; this was a private secret. I often prayed, which helped, but it would have been nice to have had a human heart to confide in. Who could I trust? This was a place where gossip got around quickly. Anxiety took hold of me and I was going to quit, but I met up with a nurse who came from Kenya. She was also a Christian and had a little boy, who was being fostered out in Leeds. We got talking and I told her about my problem and that I wanted to leave. She said I must not, because in eight months I would be qualified, and then if I passed, I would earn enough money to get home and get a good job in my own country. She was right. It was heart-breaking but I must not give up. Church-going kept me sane, and talking to my friend helped.

Examination time; I had my books out all hours, trying to cram as much as I could into my brain. I was a real bookworm. The written exam was three hours in the classroom, then the GNC exam, held in Claxon Hall in London. It was a nail-biting time. When the bell rang, you started; three hours later it rang again. During the first few minutes some people walked out, I understood that those who did, read the exam papers and did not think they could do it, so they left. I was a bit apprehensive, but felt I could answer most of the questions. Time went quickly, I thought. All was over and I was on the way to fulfilling my desire.

On the way to the hospital I was pondering the questions. I felt good, and although I did not want to disappoint myself or give myself false hope, I had studied and prepared well. Some of the nurses whom I had befriended were anxious to hear of how I had got on. I gave very little away; I did not want to give them the impression that I had done well as the results would not come for six weeks.

Next week was the hospital practical. It was held on the ward, with examiners from outside who came in to test us. Most of us did well. Time seemed to drag but I consoled myself with the thought that I would go home to see the children and my family. Money was short; I had very little in the bank. I had to think about how I would get home. Air travel was too expensive, which left travel by sea. Another chapter in my life. I made enquiries at the travel agency about dates of ships for Trinidad. There was one leaving in November. This was ideal but I had to pay for the ticket in a few days. When I checked with the bank, I did not have the full fare. What to do now? There was no loan that could help me. I prayed that the dear Lord would help me.

Next day, at breakfast, I met up with one of my coun-

The Tale of a Widow's Anguish

trymen. I told her of the problem and she said she would be able to lend me the money upfront but I had to pay it back before I left to go home. I was excited indeed. We both were on the same shift so went to the bank together, where she gave me the money. Immediately, I went to the travel agency and paid the full amount. I began to make a list to what to buy as presents to take home, because people think when someone comes home from abroad they are loaded with money.

*

Time was spinning by and I had to put my few belongings together. Of course, I had very little; mostly just books, which I would take with me because they were expensive. I would also need them to recap on things. I was to give my notice in, so I went to see Matron and told her of my plans.

An appointment was made for me to see Matron. She said I was a good nurse and I ought to wait until the results were back because I could start midwifery training when the term began. I told her the idea was good, but first I must go home. She said it was a lot of money, going and coming back. I said it was important (but I could not tell her the reason why I was leaving as I was ashamed of my past).

I told her I would like to do midwifery, as my mum had died in childbirth. She wished me all the best and told me I was most welcome to come to her hospital to further my studies if I wanted.

Well, prize giving was to be at the end of the month just before I was to leave and I was still anxiously waiting for the GNC result. Each day, when the post arrived, I

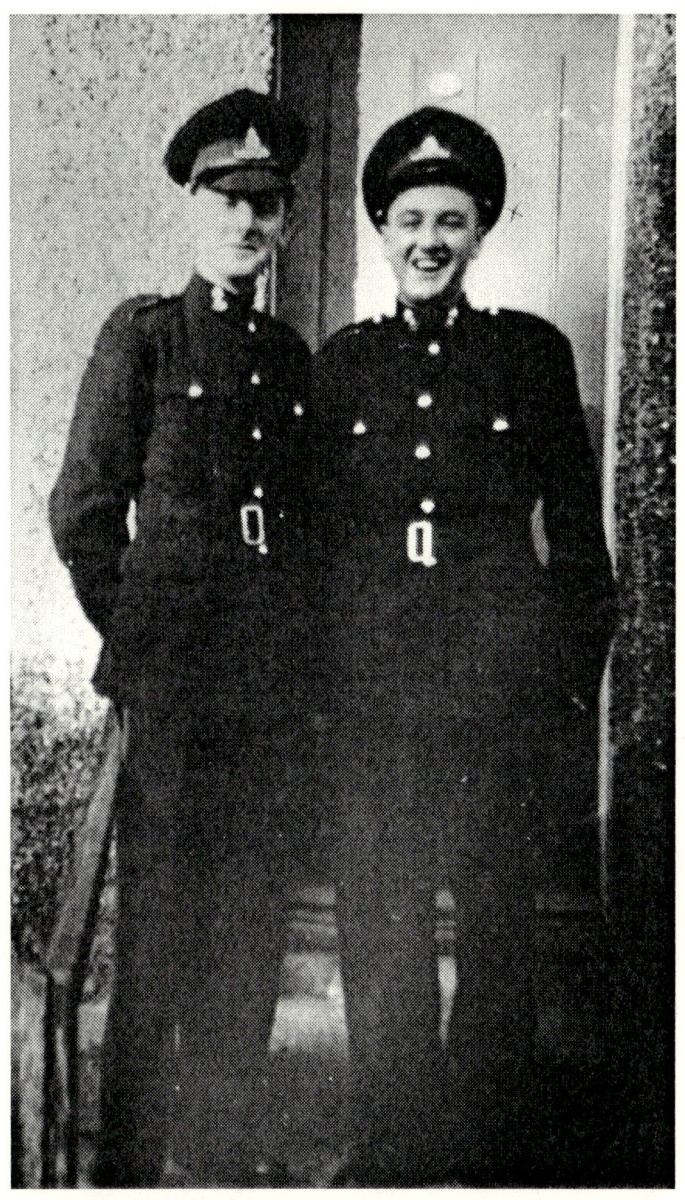

David, my husband (right) when he was in the Army, 1949

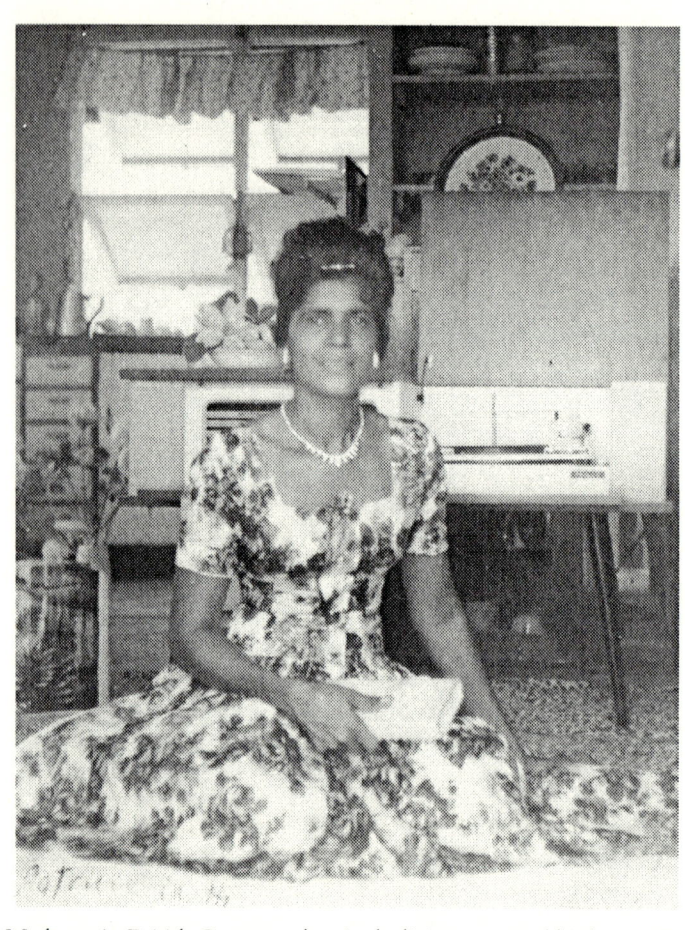

*My home in British Gayana, taken in the living room and kitchen, 1958.
I was twenty-four years old.*

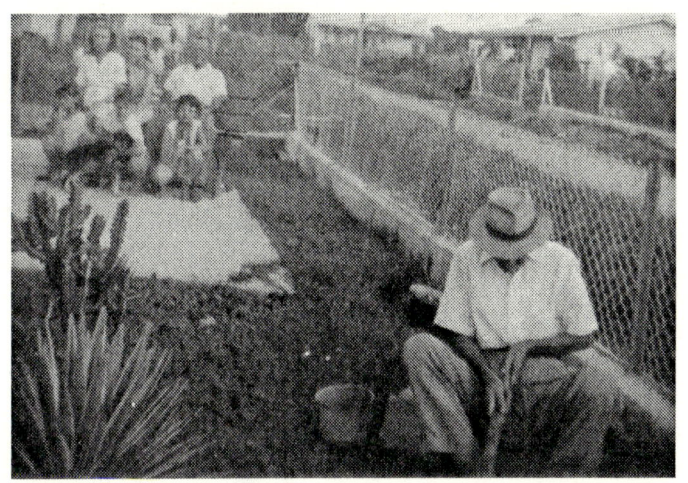

My kind neighbour's father, who helped my with the children, 1958.

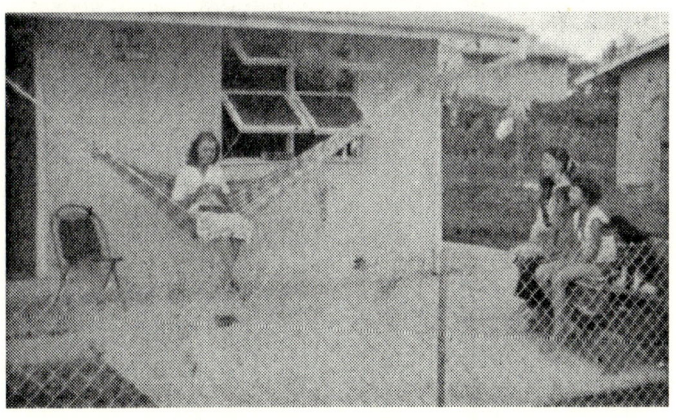

My neighbour Olage, my tower of strength.

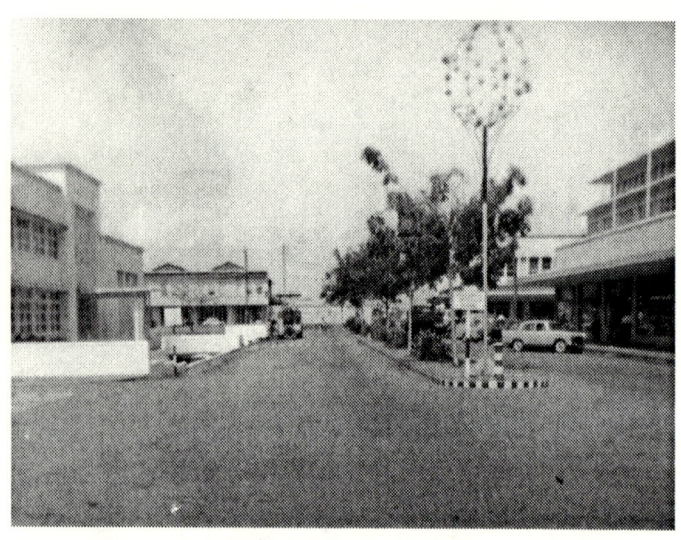

Georgetown, Guyana, 1959.

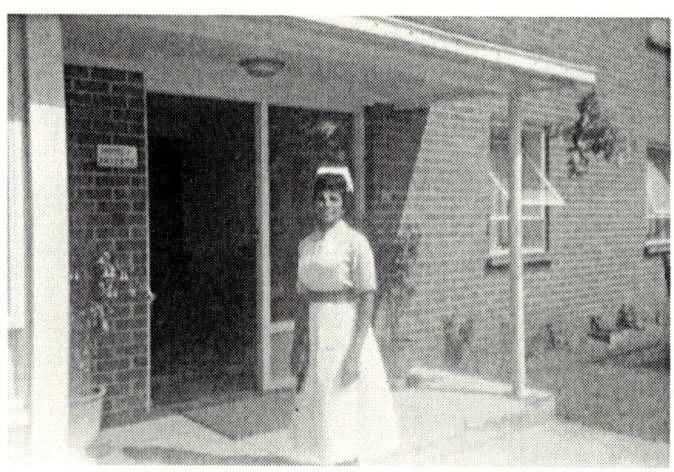

Me outside the nurses' home at Ellis Mere Hospital, Surrey, where I was training to become a nurse's aid, January/February 1964.

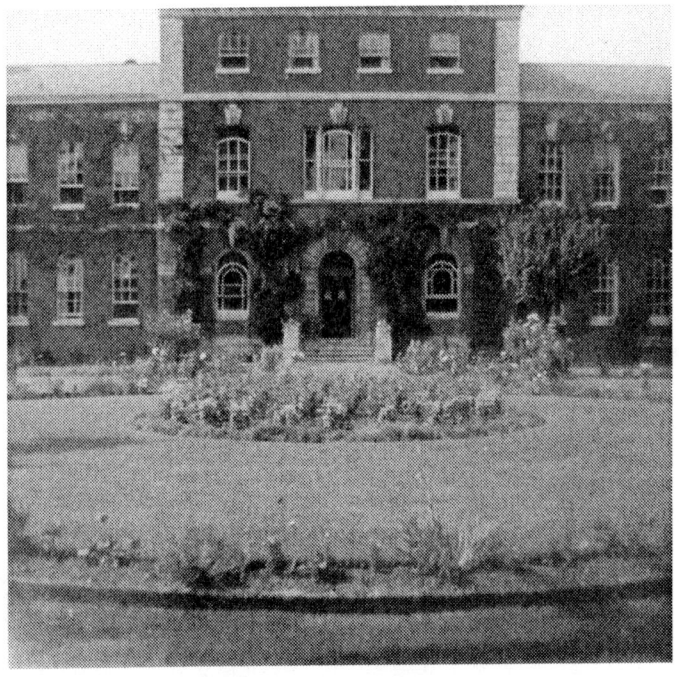

The Joyce Green Hospital, Dartford, where I did my nurse's training, 1964.

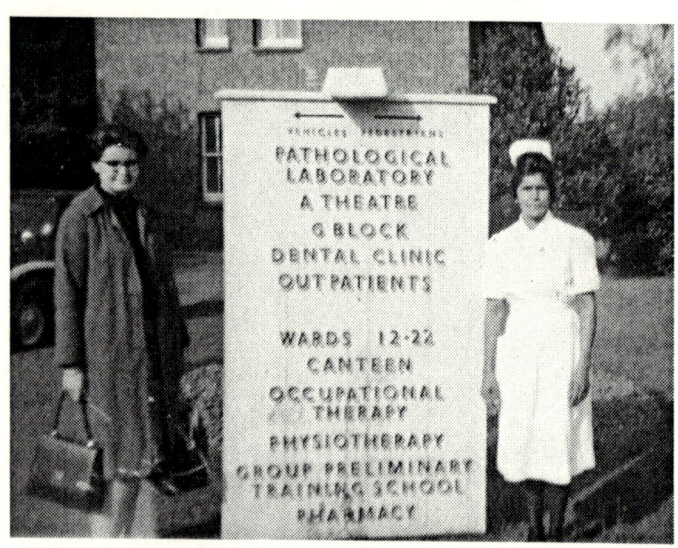

The entrance to the Joyce Green Hospital. Kathy Kennedy, who lived in Bromley, Kent, left, and myself.

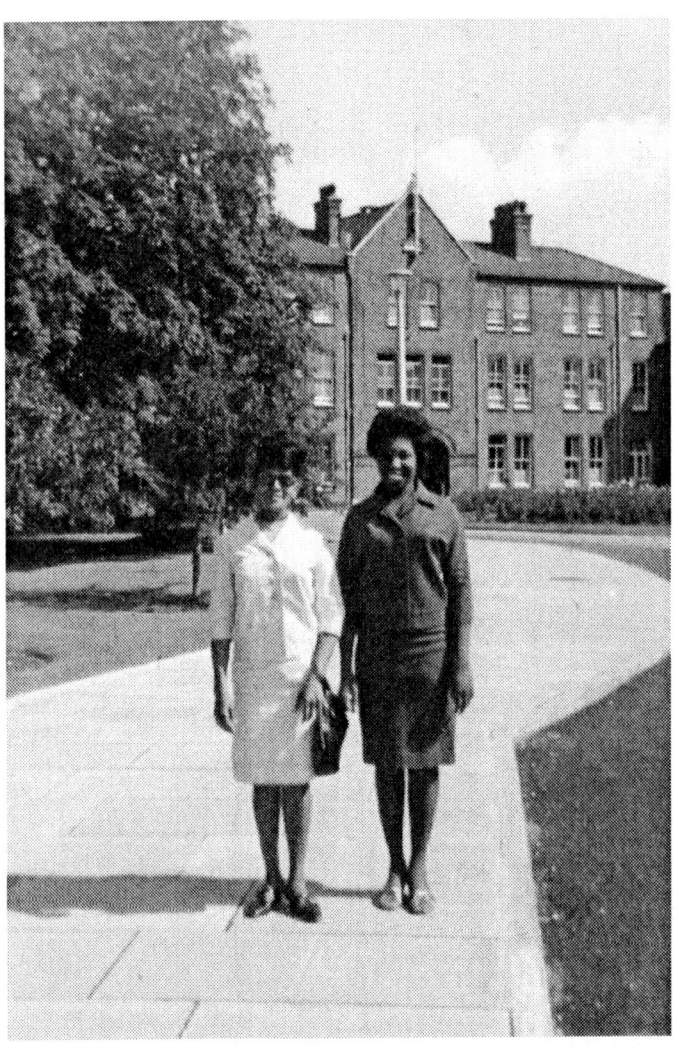
Joyce Green Hospital. Me on the left with my friend, Artelene Williams.

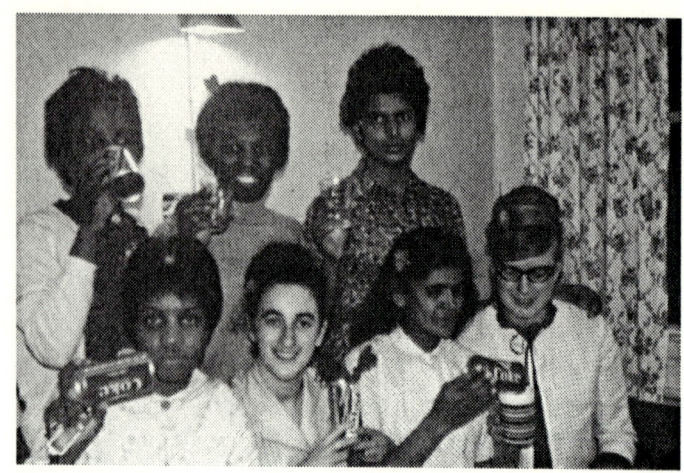

Top row, from left: Pribor from Sri Lanka; Masa from Barbados; Artelene from Guyana. Bottom row, from left: unknown; Evid from Sweden; me with a red rose in my hair; Barbara from Manchester, having a Christian Coke party at Joyce Green Hospital in the late 1960s.

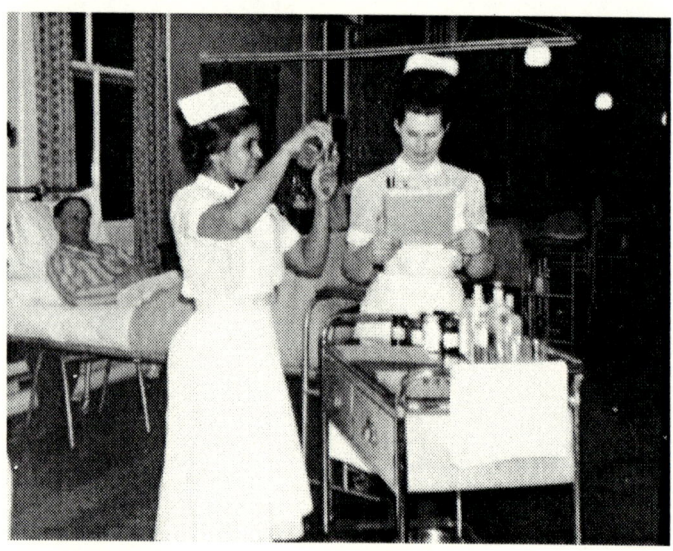

Me doing the drug round on the ward with Maureen O'Flauty and the patient Mr Dorsey at the Joyce Green Hospital, 1964/5.

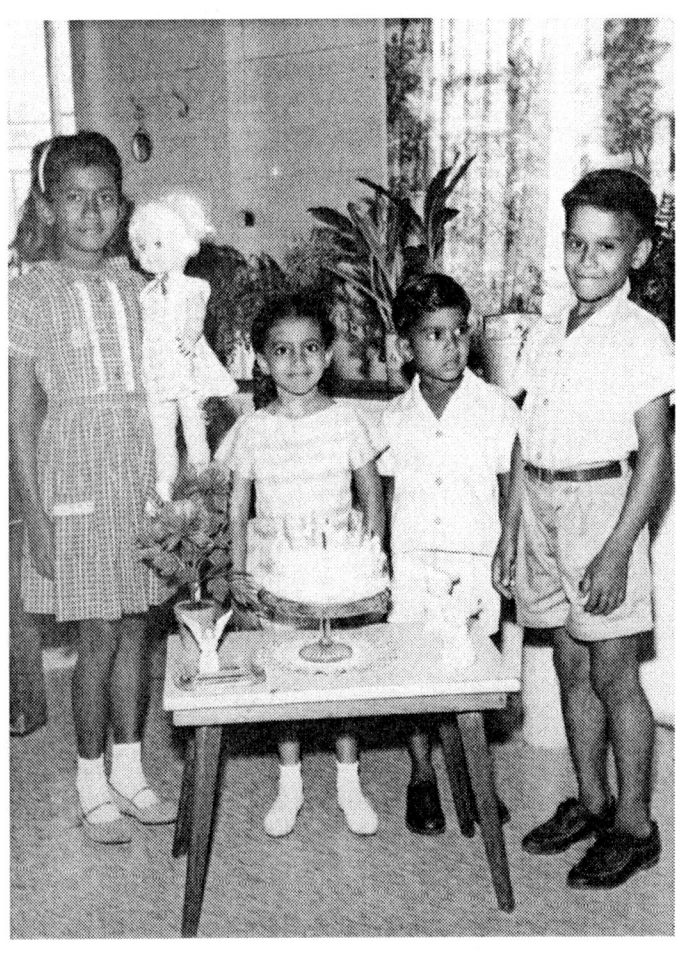

From left to right: Babs, ten; Tom, four; Jo, eight; and their cousin, Guyana.

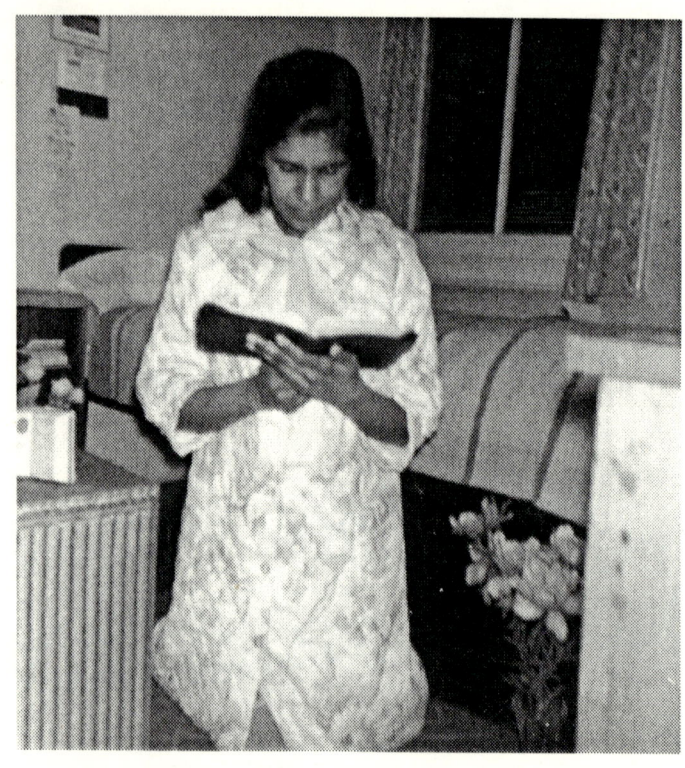

Me, reading my bible in my little room in the nurses' home. It was so small there was only just space to move about, 1964.

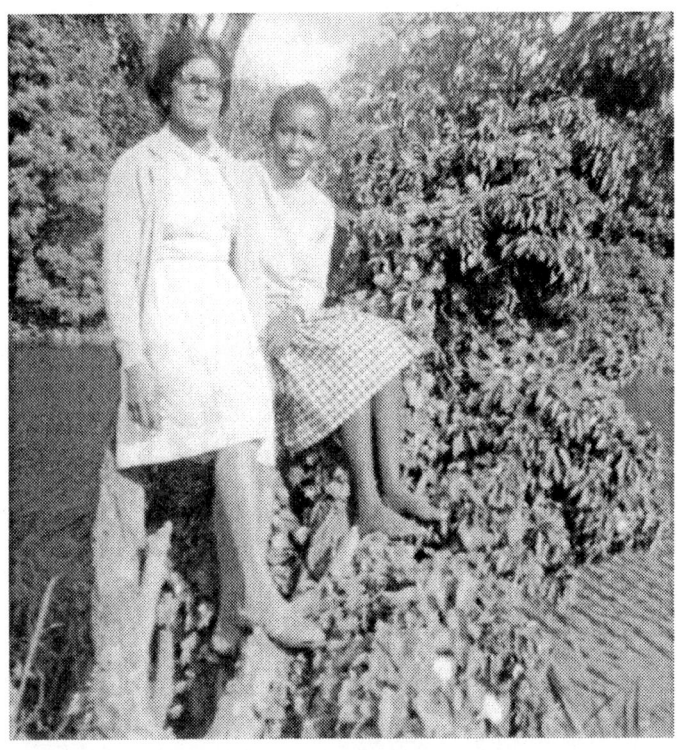

Me and Jerusha, my best friend, climbing a tree while picnicking. Jerusha returned to Kenya with her little boy, never to be seen again.

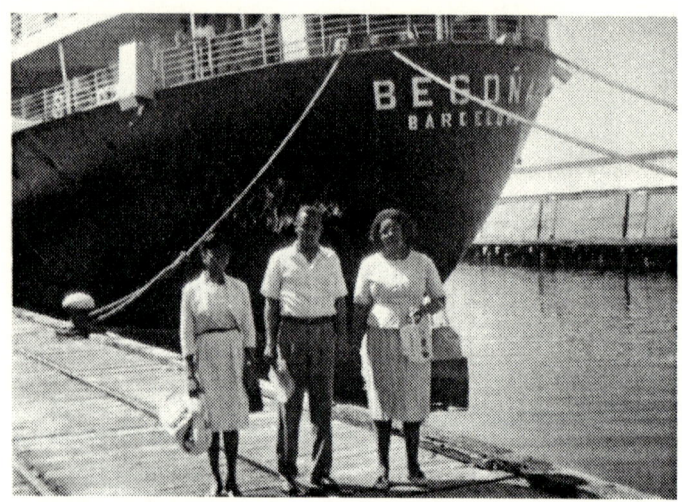

From left to right: me; Collin and Jack's wife, Norma, going back to Guyana after completing training, 1966.

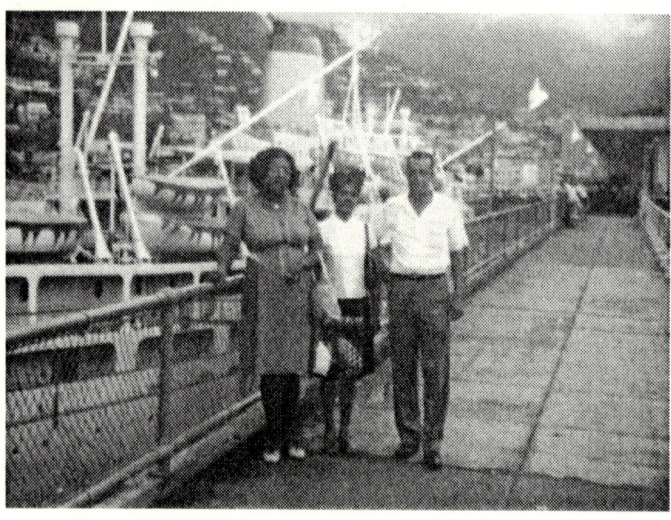

Getting off the boat at Barcelona, 1966. From left to right: Norma; me; Collin.

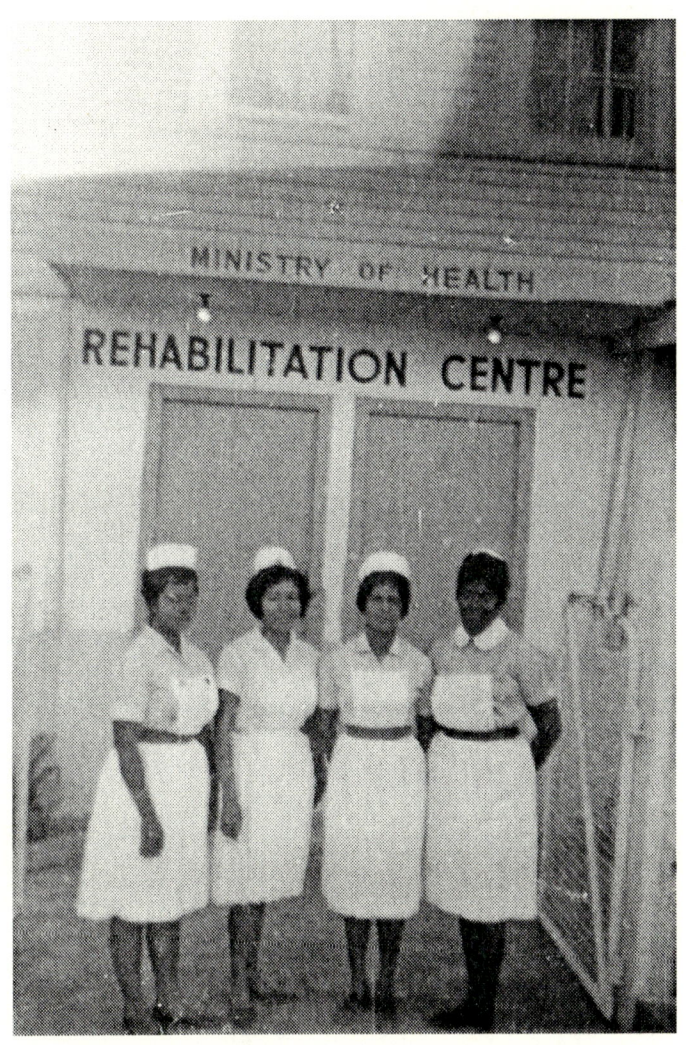

A rehabilitation centre for children suffering from polio in Guyana, where I worked for six months in 1967.

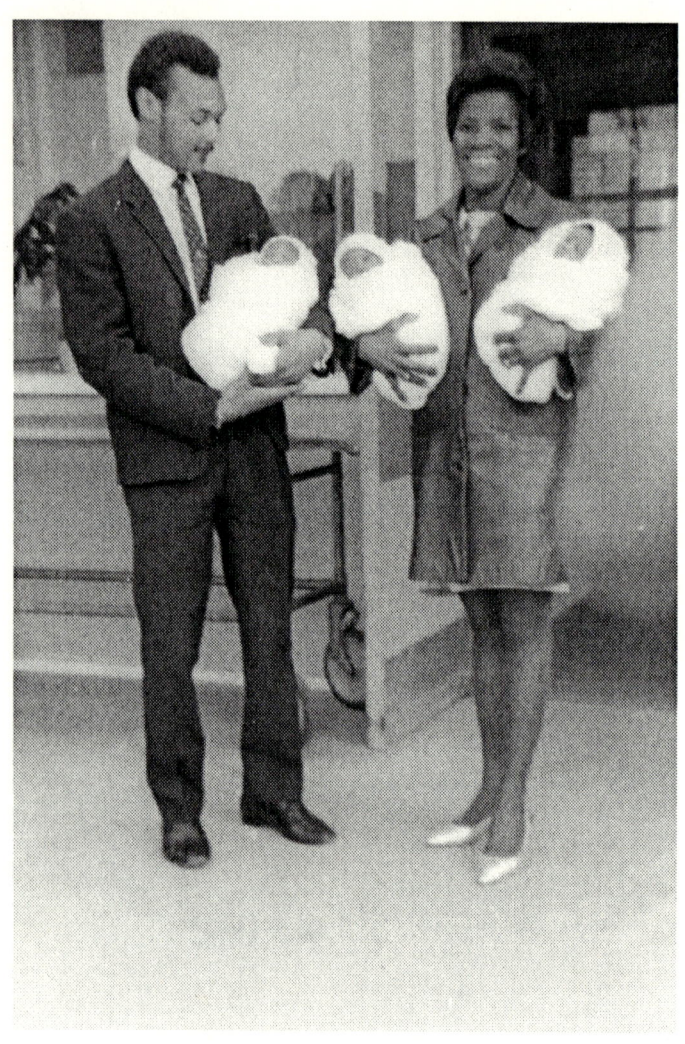

Quads that I looked after at Rochford Maternity Hospital in Essex, 1969.

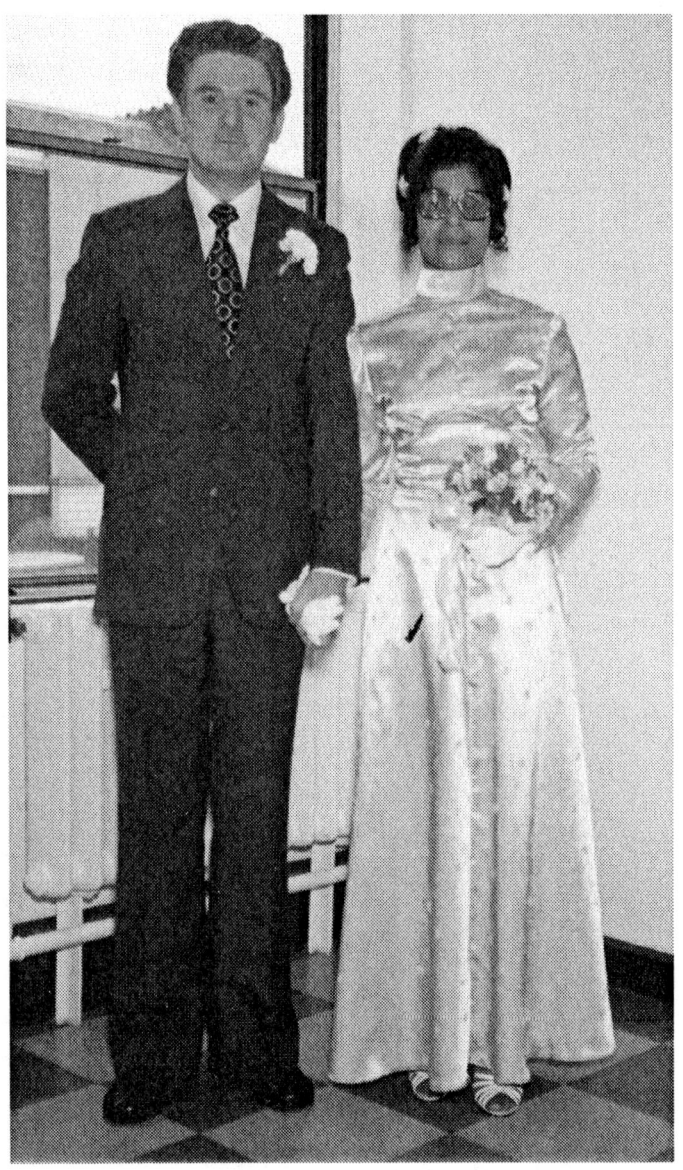

My wedding to Mr David John Deamer at Gravesend Registry Office, 21 May 1976.

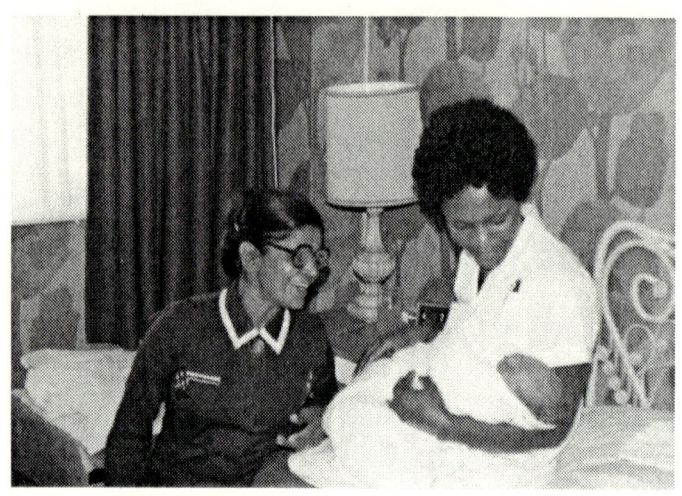

A home delivery in Kent, 1977.

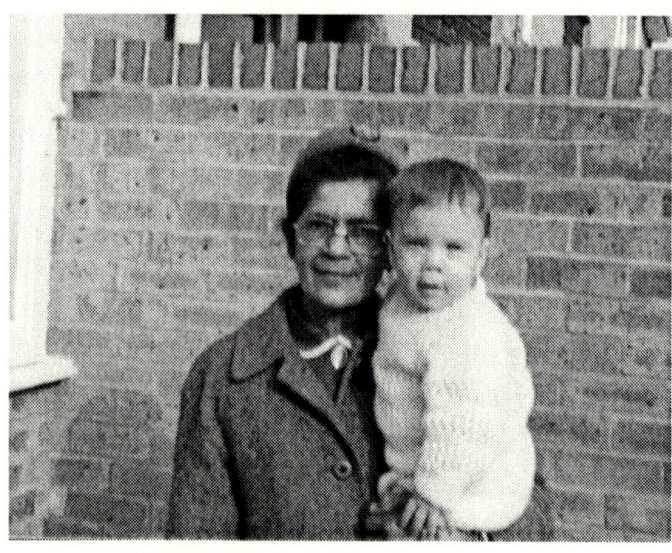

One of the babies I delivered, spring 1984.

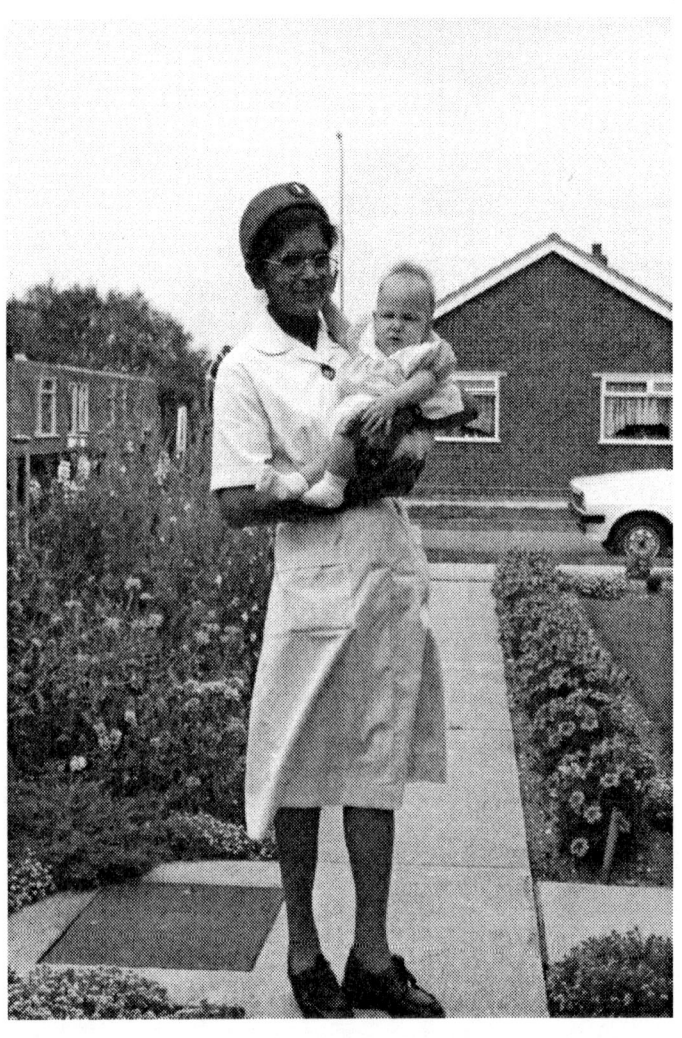

Debbie Anne Fitzpatrick, one of the babies I delivered while a midwife in 1981.

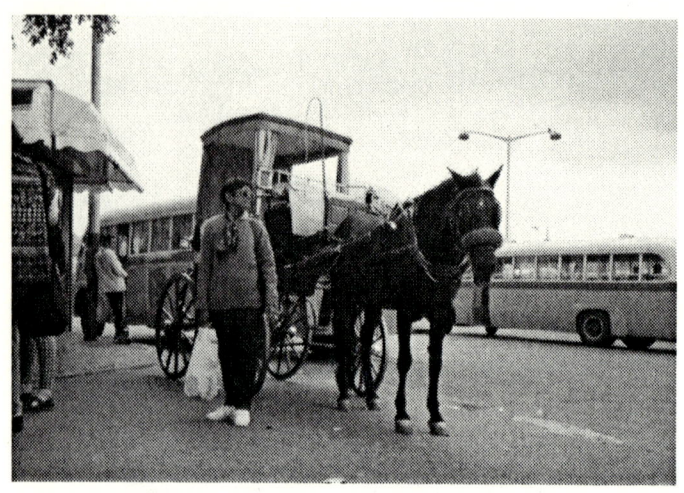

Me at Valetta bus depot in Malta, 1997.

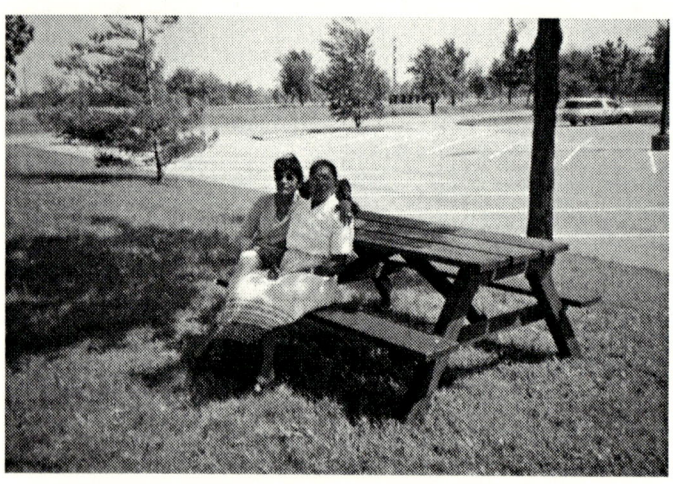

With my sister Ree, taken in Canada five years ago.

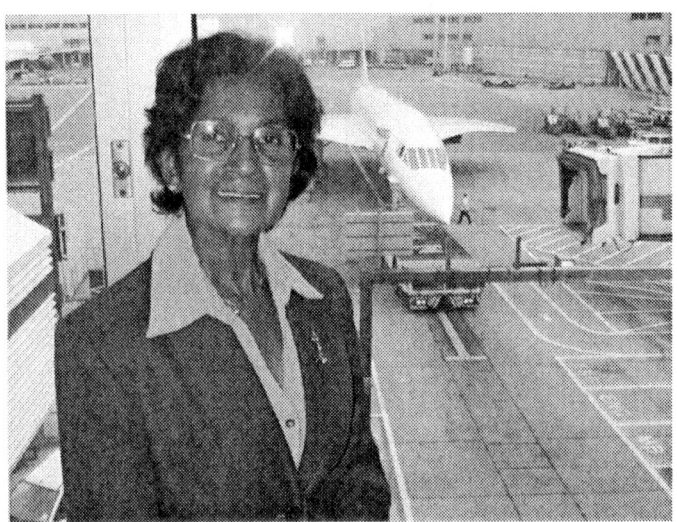

Flying on Concorde on 3 September 2003, London Heathrow to JFK New York.

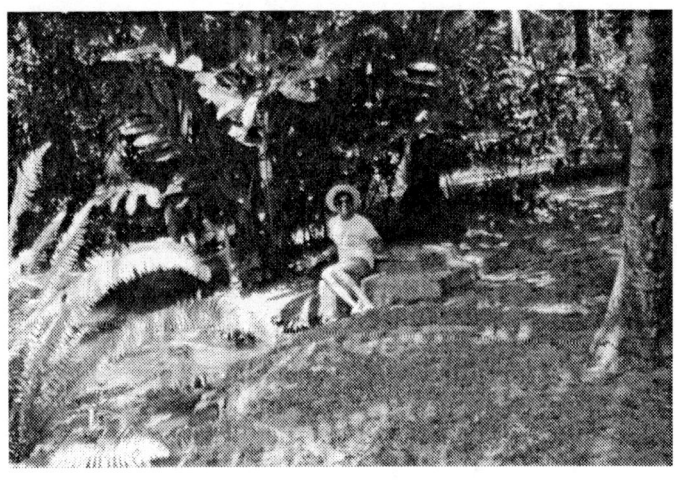

Me at Durun's Waterfall, with ginger lilies at the sides.

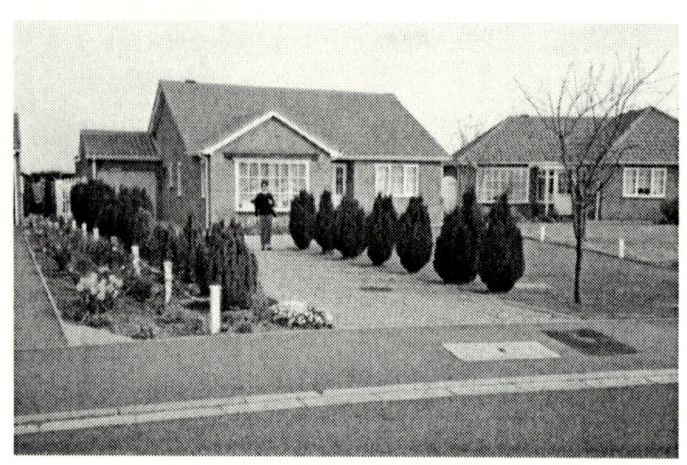

Me outside my last home in Headington.

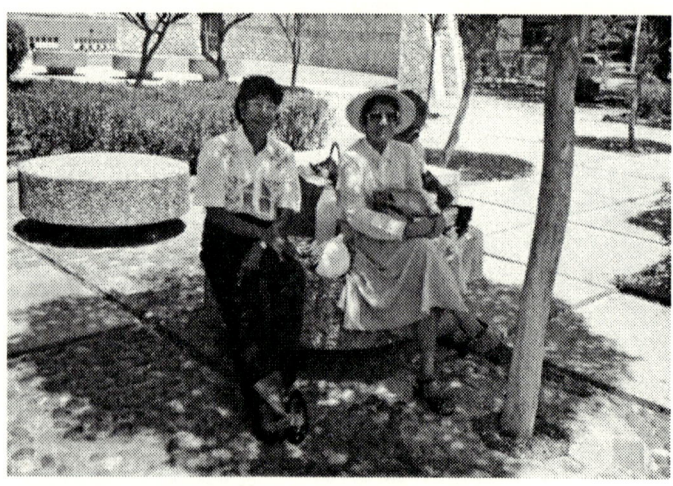

With my favourite niece, Evelyn Pat Rita, picnicking in Jamaica.

would check the pigeonhole to see if a brown envelope had arrived for me. My heart would be pounding away. I was full of anxious thoughts; if the result came and I had failed, what would happen?

Notice was given. My gratuity pay was in the bank, my ticket had arrived and I had been awarded the tutor's prize – a good English dictionary, which I had wanted but was unable to buy, and a hymnbook, which I was glad to receive. I was sad to leave but had important things to sort out when I got home. The night before I left, a little party was held by the friends I had made. Some shed a few tears, wishing it was them going home. If they only knew the torment I was going through in my head, living in fear of John and his family.

I thought the God who brought me through so far would see me through this trauma and work something out for me. I resolved to go back to John when I returned, to tell him I was sorry and ask if we could get together for the children's sake. My friend took me to Waterloo station, where I went on the main line to Southampton, where I joined the Spanish ship. In my cabin was one other lady who was going to Jamaica. She seemed pushy and wanted to have her own way. I was bullied all the time. Courage, I told myself; I am not a doormat for everyone to walk on.

*

We were off and I felt wonderful. I met lots of people who were going back from holiday and I talked to those who were eager to share the time they had and the experiences they had gained. I was happy for them. One couple knew my brother-in-law. While talking to me, the husband said he was the manager of the roadworks department and was delighted to meet me. We all settled in and enjoyed the sailing, particularly when the ship stopped, in the same manner as it did when I first went to the UK. I was more relaxed then on my outward journey.

Miss Bossy was tipsy one evening and I went early to my cabin. She came in and said someone had stolen her money. I asked her how this could happen because it was only the two of us in the cabin; I told her my money was in the ship safe and I only had a few pounds on me. I advised her to report the matter to the officer in charge. Well, the next day, she said she had found the money; she had misplaced it. I suggested she keep it in the safe from now on. I was unhappy, as I felt she had accused me of stealing. However, when we landed at her port, I gave her a hearty goodbye.

Time was getting on and the sea was becoming a bit restless; some of us developed sea-sickness. As for me, being a nurse, I had all the pills for most things, which I shared with those who complained of minor ailments. I was glad to be of some help, although they had a hospital nurse on board the ship.

I prayed all the time when I was alone for God to keep me safe, to help me make the right decisions and that I would get good news about my exam.

I met up with a nice man on his own. He seemed quite a charmer and for the first time I fancied someone. He seemed a gentleman, and we chatted about our country and how things were not the same as when the Brits ruled. While I was away my country had gained independence and the people were now fighting each other, so he said. I told him I was about to be qualified as a registered nurse. He was pleased for me and said there was plenty of work for people like me. He asked for my address but I declined because my family would not have taken kindly to him. However, I told him perhaps one day we'd meet again.

*

The ship docked. I stayed overnight at a hotel and the next day I made my way to the airport, through customs and onto the plane. At take-off time, I had mixed feelings as to what I was doing. I was very nervous as we landed. My dad and a few people came to meet me with big hugs and kisses from my sister. When we arrived at my sister's home, it was late afternoon and none of my children were in sight. I asked for them; the bombshell dropped John's mother had come and collected the three of them four weeks ago.

I think the news had got out that I was returning home and this was when the trouble began. However, whatever happened, I would fight to have my children back. I made plans to see them at the weekend and asked for some back-up. My sister would have to come with me.

*

Next morning, the postman arrived and there was a brown envelope given to me. I was so pleased but nervous to open it. My sister sensed that I had something important in the envelope. I said to her it was the exam result; she thought that I had got the result before leaving the UK. I opened it carefully and to my delight I had passed. I praised the Lord and was so happy to have some

The Tale of a Widow's Anguish

good thing happen in my life. I could get a job now; I would write to all the hospitals – private establishments as well.

But I had to get those children, no matter what the cost. My brother-in-law was away, and this was in my favour.

A cousin came to welcome me home and asked where my new husband was. I was dumfounded at this remark. Gossip had gone around that I had left the country with another man. I did not have time to explain; I just ignored him. He said I must not visit any of my family because I had caused disgrace to them, as no one ever left their husband and children and went away for three years.

End of story, I said, and went. As it was the weekend, my sister and I went to see the children. They seemed OK. Babs was very tearful; the two boys were aloof but hugs and kisses were exchanged. Mother-in-law, Jess, was quiet, but said if I had to stay, I would have to abide by the rules of the house and that the children would not leave. I had to make a decision now. I thought I would give it a try; staying in the town would help me secure a job. And a private hospital was only walking distance away.

*

My sister, Ree, advised caution. Jess said she only had the sitting room so I could put a bed in the corner and a curtain could act as a screen for my privacy. I took up the offer and promised to pay for my lodging. Later that afternoon, to my surprise, Jene, my stepsister, arrived with lots of smiles. Jess, it appeared, had gone to the market as she had lots of vegetables and fishes in her basket. This was given to Babs to put away. I went to my so-called room and the three children came along with me. I handed out a few presents, but had none for the others. Jene was upset; she asked why I came back and said that John and her were living together and the children were happy with that arrangement. I was furious but kept cool, telling myself to let sleeping dogs lie – a wise saying.

I was given a mattress, which was placed on the floor and a few other things as all my belongings were left at Ree's house. The children slept in one room and the rest were rented out to lodgers. Jene and John had a room for themselves. This was a real nightmare and I had to take action soon. I didn't like this set-up at all, but I went along with whatever was thrown at me.

I made a visit to the private hospital and asked to see the Matron. She was nice, but said they only employed Christians to work there, as it was a missionary hospital. I emphasised that I was a churchgoer and that I could get a reference from my pastor in the UK. She took details and said I would hear from her. I was delighted, and went back to my little dwelling to tell Babs that I would soon have a job.

I went to see my sister to talk about what was best to do if I moved away and was cut off from the children. We talked about custody of the children and what action I could take. We had little idea though, and I went back home – if I could call it home at all. John was about but we did not cross paths. I tried to avoid him and Jene and Jess did all the bullying and talking. They treated me with contempt always, saying I was not wanted. Oh, how this ached my heart. I wished to escape with the children.

The Tale of a Widow's Anguish

I received news that I had a job. The pay was good but I must attend their church. I went when I was not working. Before we commenced shift, prayer was said and all the wards had an intercom for the patients to listen in. It was a wonderful experience to work there. We got our meals provided; all vegetarian dishes. Tasty.

Three months later, I went to see the Matron at the Government hospital and asked if there was a course on midwifery; there was, but there was also a waiting list, as usual, of a year. I was offered a job working on the obstetric unit until the take-in time. I went to see my sister and told her that if she did not mind me staying with her, I could get a job in this other hospital and move out of enemy quarters. OK, she said, but how would I be able to persuade John that it would be good for the children to come and live with me? I applied for the job and rented a place in the town and tried and see the children as often as possible.

*

Blackmail began. John said to me if I slept with him for a while I could move out and take the children; I refused. Well, he gave me such a shake that I fell over, and went tumbling down the stairs. Jess came along and said to just kill me. It was devastating. I went and talked to the man next door, who was a shopkeeper. He said they were a mixed up family and that he, John, had VD, and all the women he was sleeping with had to go for treatment.

Well, I waited for the children to come home and told them I would be away for a few days. I told Matron of the episode and she said I would have to get somewhere safe to stay because of my work. I went away for one night only and met up with the children; each night I got a place to stay nearby. But my life was threatened, and so other plans had to be made. John would come to the hospital looking for me; I had to warn the porter, saying that he was waiting to harm me. I had to get out through the back gate, which said 'no exit'. Terrifying indeed.

I had to move out. My name was on the waiting list at the other hospital, and I was called for the post as Matron had promised. I told the children but they were to keep it as a secret.

We met up and had meals out at a place called Brown Betty in the town; lots of ice cream, which the children enjoyed. I started my new job, which I hated because we were so short of nurses. However, my enemies soon found out where I was working and I was back to square one.

Jene was the one who came to haunt me. She hated me so much because I had a career and she was a home help for Jess and her son. I went to church regularly and met some honest people I could talk to and the minister was a real friend. He would ask me to bring the children over and have meals with him and his family. We went a few times but did not make it a habit. I would take baskets of fruit to say thank you.

Changes must be made, I thought. I would ask the minister what he thought, and so I told him about my plans. He said that if it was possible, I could go back to the UK and send for the children, if I could get custody of them. He promised to pray for me.

I had a visitor waiting for me when I got off work. Lo and behold, it was John's brother, Neil. I was a bit anxious to know why he had come to see me, He said hello and asked how I was. I was very antisocial for a moment then asked why he was there. He said quietly that I must leave the country and send for the children and that he would help me to get them out. He knew a good solicitor who would write letters to the British Embassy. I was cautious, not saying yes or no. I wanted to know why he was keen to help me and was not taking his brother's side. He said John and Jene were both suffering from some nasty disease and they would try to give it to me. He complimented me on getting a career and left me confused.

Well, I did not know what to believe. When I was off, I went to see Ree and my dad was there. I told them about my visitor. Dad was on the defensive about Jene, and said he could not give account for her actions now she was of age; and as for John, he did sleep with lots of women. I was angry and did not say I wanted to leave the country. He went and I told Ree how I was scared out of my mind and could not bear to spend the rest of my life living in fear. She said I had to consider what was best for me. I thought that life was a circle, and by God's help, a way of escape would be. Oh, how I prayed.

I would not give up; I would not let my enemies triumph over me. I went to the travel agencies and asked about the cost of a single adult fare to Britain, and singles for the three children. I could afford it; money was in the bank as I was a good saver. I went to the British Consulate and told them I would like a student visa to study midwifery, and took all my papers to prove that I was a qualified nurse. The same day, I got my passport stamped with a student visa.

Flight booked, notice given to quit my job, I waited until I was ready to fly out of the country. I only told Babs of my plans and how sorry I was to leave them again but that I would send for them as soon as possible. I visited the school and told the headmistress of my plans. She said the youngest had learning difficulties and that she had sent a letter asking John to come and see her regarding Tom's problem. However, she said she would get someone to give him special attention.

It was time to make contact with Matron to tell her I was coming back to further my studies, and Sarah, the friend I used to stay with. It was easy. Neil visited frequently. He seemed genuine and I started to trust him, but did not say too much just in case there was a trap.

*

It was time for me to leave. I took the children to see Ree, as it was the weekend. I told them the situation; it was a sad time for all of us. Parting is awful. But we would meet again; after all, God was with me. I had to be brave. It was the weekend and the flight was at night; a good time to escape. I told Neil I would be away for a while and if he needed to contact me it could be done through my sister.

At the airport, I said a tearful goodbye to my children. It was harder this time as they were growing up and I felt my world was caving in. At Heathrow, a few friends from the church came to fetch me. I spent a few days with them, and told them about the children. Their faces dropped. Some shed a few tears, saying what an ordeal I was going through. Some offered to keep me.

I took up one offer, which was near the hospital, and contacted Matron, to get a date when I could see her. During this time, I was making plans to get the children over. I was told I could start training at the beginning of the month and could live in if I wanted to. I was glad to and settled in nicely. When I was off I visited estate agencies asking how I could buy a house. I was told about down payments and how a mortgage could be set up. I visited schools to see if they would take the children. I found several, and I put their names down on the register to hold the place. Three months had passed and I was making progress and receiving letters from Ree. But then I got one from Neil, saying his mum did not want the children. I cried so much I wished I was dead.

I wrote to the Home Office asking them to give me a resident visa, as I wanted to live and work in the UK when I was qualified. Eventually I received a letter from the Home Office granting me indefinite leave to remain. Well, this was good news; the children had visas to come and live with me, so I had to get a home for us to live in and then send their tickets. I needed a lot of money to do this. I had money, but not to do all this in one go. However, I sent the flight tickets for the children, and made arrangements to buy a two-bedroom house. It was a mid-terrace, costing £3,500, well decorated. An old couple was moving. They left lots of curtains and bits for me. I had to borrow £300 for the down payment. When I was qualified I would pay my friend back with some interest. Life was very hectic and I was halfway through my training. I had to shop to get the children warm clothing, as it was winter now and they would feel the cold. Everything was under control and the children were to arrive the next day at Gatwick airport.

I knew the time of arrival, and as I was off duty I took the train to Charing Cross and another to Gatwick. I waited for three hours; no one turned up. I made enquiries about why they were not on the flight. The lady at the airline desk said I should contact the agency where the ticket was bought. Luckily, I had my diary with me. I made a few phone calls, but my money was running out. I set off home disappointed indeed. I got home and tried to call Neil at his work place. He said he was sorry. I told him this waiting game was costing me money. He replied that John had stopped the children from going to the airport. I was mad and burst into tears. He said there was a flight leaving next week and he would see that they got on the flight. I did not believe him and became convinced it was a set up. I rang a friend and she said all would be well. I went to bed, as it was late evening, but I was unable to sleep.

Later that week, Neil called with the date and time the children would arrive at Gatwick. I managed to get the day off, switching with a colleague. I was all set for my trip to the airport. After much changing of trains, I arrived, with a half-hour to go. I waited at Arrivals, chewing on some peanuts I'd bought; an anxious time for me. Suddenly, I saw the three of them holding hands making their way towards the exit. I was so excited, and shouted their names, waving like mad. Lots of hugs and kisses and a few tears. I helped with putting their coats on and offered to buy some food. But they were too excited and wanted us to get home.

We got home late. I fed them and got them ready for bed. They did not have many clothes and no pocket money. I told them not to worry, we would make do with what we had. I had the heater on all night because it was cold and coming from a hot climate they would feel the cold. The next day I had to go to work, but I had the weekend off, as well as a week's holiday. I gave them instructions what to do and where things were kept so

The Tale of a Widow's Anguish

they would find it easy to adapt. I told them they had to go to school, that it was not far from home – within walking distance – and that I would take them on the first day.

Monday morning came and they dressed, looking very smart in their uniforms, matching blazers and coats, which cost me a lot of money. It was worth the trouble. I had a lot to do and think about; my exams were quite soon and I would have to do some hard studying, as I was the only bread-winner. We had no TV but lots of games and second-hand puzzles I had bought for them. My neighbour next door was kind and she had two boys who made friends with my two. Babs went to the town and got to know the place, I took them to the park and told them the rules: to tidy their rooms up and help to make life easy, as I was very busy and needed their cooperation. We were making good progress and it was time for my big examination. I was more relaxed this time as I had the children and a career ahead. That week I did the written, and a week later, the practical at Middlesex Hospital. I was confident that I would pass the exam. Weeks went by before I learned that I had passed. Oh, it was a joy! I told my neighbour, Eileen. She went and got us a bottle of ginger wine and some squash for the children. News had to reach my sister; I wrote her a letter of my success. I praised the Lord and told all my friends of the good news.

The children were well behaved and ate anything I put at the table. We attended church every Sunday, but I felt odd because I did not have a husband and the children had no father; I was really embarrassed when anyone asked about the children's father. I would say it was a long story and I would tell them in due course. I told the children if anyone asked where was their father, just to say he was back home and don't answer any more questions. It was a taboo in those days, not having a husband. I held my head up high and tried to ignore those who disapproved of me.

I earned more now, but had to meet more financial demands. I bought bare necessities: cheap cuts of meat, plenty of vegetables, potatoes, oats for breakfast; we could not afford to buy any packaged food. The children were content and did not grumble too much. They would not, as I had already told them we were struggling to cope.

There was a post going in the district, but you had to hold a driving licence and I did not have one. I spoke to a friend of mine who said the NHS would pay for lessons and the test but I would have to sign a contract for two years; this was what I was looking for. I wrote to County Hall and asked for an application form. I completed it and then sent it, along with names of references. I discussed the situation with my children and they approved.

The only drawback was that it meant antisocial hours and more weekend work. We would have to cope somehow. Babs was good with Tom but Jo was a bit moody sometimes. I told him to try and cooperate and life would get better; we would be able to go out to the seaside when the summer came as a car would be provided with the new job.

*

Climbing the ladder now, I got the job, and earned more money but it meant lots of night calls. I had to take a taxi to the patient's home, although sometimes the husband would come to collect me, for which I was grateful.

The Tale of a Widow's Anguish

It was not easy. I had to snatch some sleep when I was alone because when the boys got home they were a bit noisy. Babs would take control; she was good with them. Life was hectic but I had a lot of energy. Work; housework; learning to drive; gardening; making clothes for the children (or to the second-hand shop). Babs would not wear second-hand clothes; she rebelled. I told her if she wanted new ones, she would have to do a paper-round to get some money.

I took my driving test and failed. I was very wound up before the test but the instructor was kind and said I could put in for another test right away. I was so sad and thought I would never make it. We called a meeting at tea time, the four of us. Over tea I said to them I would go back to the hospital to work, because things were getting me down. You should have seen their faces; all three were about to cry. They all told me to have another go. I agreed to try again – just one more time; then if I failed I would quit. More lessons and a test after a few weeks. My contract gave me one year to pass the test; if not, I would lose the job. I really wanted that job, as it came with a car and private mileage. Yes, I had to try, and take a few more lessons; if it meant going over the budget I would foot the bill, as long as I passed. Lots of prayers were said at the church for me, That night I prayed that God might hear my request.

I never believed in gipsy curses, but the next morning was my test and there came a knock on my door. A lady was there with a basket, selling tit-bits. I had a few shillings only, but as the saying goes, if you do not buy from a gipsy, she will curse you. I bought something which I cannot remember now, but a great smile came on her face. She gave me a small horseshoe and said I would have good luck. I thought it was garbage; I had to earn my crust and trust God for all my needs.

I had a cup of tea and went for the driving test. I passed with flying colours, so maybe the gypsy lady was right. I don't know. Well, I had good news for the children. As it was my weekend off, I thought we'd have a little party to celebrate. We had a few cakes and orange drink with Eileen and her two sons. We sang and made a bit of noise. It was wonderful indeed; I was fully qualified. Now I could pay my friend the loan back and could take the children places. I signed a full contract at County Hall and a blue Mini car was issued, with instructions as to where to get petrol. This was exactly what I needed.

*

No stopping me now! But then a huge electricity bill came in, and other utility bills at the same time. My mortgage went up; there were stratospheric interest rates – this was in the Seventies – but I would cope with good budgeting. I was a careful manager.

Summer arrived and I took the children out in the car. We went to the seaside for a day out. Carrying our own refreshment to save money, we all had great fun. It was a happy time for me and no looking back any more.

*

The children were growing up fast and, unfortunately, Tom had to go to a special school, because of his learning difficulties. He was not so happy, but I encouraged him to do his best.

Babs was sixteen now, saying she wanted to leave school and find a job. I told her she should go for a career

The Tale of a Widow's Anguish

as it would pay off when she got older. She left school and got a job as a junior clerk, earning her own money. I spoke to her, asking if she could put some money towards the food, as the boys needed more pocket money, and clothing was expensive and there were bills to pay. She gave me a few shillings. Most of her money went on buying clothes and make-up. She made friends and went out some evenings. I gave orders not to stay out late at night. All was not so well. She wanted a room for herself. I made one of the downstairs room into a bedroom and used the dining room for a bedroom. A few months later an old friend asked to stay with us; it was the same friend who had given me the loan.

I told her we had no room but she pleaded until I agreed to let her stay for a short while. I told her we would have to get single bed and as I had no money she would have to foot the bill. We got a second-hand bed. Babs said she would share her room because I was on call most nights. I discussed the situation with my friend. She told me she had nowhere to go as her husband had thrown her out.

What a new dilemma I was faced with! I was trapped as I had to pay this lady back her money as soon as possible. I went and saw the bank manager about a loan. He said if the money was paid back in a short time it would not cost so much. I wrote to Ree asking her to lend me the money or if she couldn't, to ask Dad to lend it to me. I said that I was desperate for the cash.

A banker's draft arrived for the necessary amount. I put it in the bank and told my friend to find a place and I would give her the money I had borrowed, along with interest. She said no and we had a big ding-dong. She had a charming nephew whom I had met a few times.

She called him on the phone to say he must come and gave directions to get to my place. He arrived and I told the two boys to go upstairs to their room, as I had visitors. She said to her nephew that she had lent me some money for the deposit of this house and because of this, she could stay with me any time she liked. Any time she liked! I was speechless. I took courage and sent the nephew packing. Before he left, he said that we could be good friends; I could be his mistress. Not over my dead body! I called him a few names, and sent him on his way.

I felt miserable. I would get a solicitor to certify that I had repaid the money, otherwise I could be the subject of a witch hunt. I felt thoroughly fed-up.

Next day, we went to town. I got a banker's draft for the full amount to pay my friend, then to a solicitor who saw the handing-over of the money and an official receipt was given to me, which costs me a few pounds. A few weeks later we found a place for her. I went with her to say our goodbyes. I came home mentally exhausted.

Babs was sulking, asking why I had to tell my friend to leave as she did not mind sharing her room. I told her I could not afford to keep five of us, as this friend did not have a job, and was not able to contribute to anything. Babs got very rude, asking if that was how I treated friends: she, Babs, gave very little money towards her keep. I told her we had had a hard time and now we must pull together; she could further her education and do nursing, or whatever she wished. Her answer was that she was leaving home to go and live with my friend and would find a job somewhere. She gave her notice and left home. Oh, how I begged her not to go; she was not streetwise and London was no place for young girls,

It all fell on deaf ears. I went ballistic and took her

passport away. She said she had to have it. 'Call the police,' I said. 'I shall send you back home!' She left as if she had no feeling for her brothers. I never figured out what was happening in her head. I would find it hard to live without her; what would I tell the boys when they came home? My world came tumbling down. I kept blaming myself, saying I had put my career before my children. I told the boys what had happened. Jo said that it was one less to feed. Tom was sad and ate little and we all went early to bed. Unable to sleep, I was wracked with guilt. Well, things can't get any worse, I consoled myself.

I wrote home to give Ree the news and on the same morning I received a letter from Ree saying John had died and Jene had gone to live in the West Indies. I was not sad at all and planned to tell the boys after tea.

I tried to contact Babs to let her know that her father had passed away. After tea, I broke the news to the boys. They did not seem to worry too much, as he didn't have their affection. I continued to work hard as usual, but Jo helped with tidying-up. Tom had his ups and downs and was getting difficult to handle.

We had a quiet Christmas, and when I was off, we went out in the woods picking bark, as I was doing flower-arranging. The bluebells were out so we gathered a few bunches for Eileen and ourselves. We made the best of life, but I always wondered what Babs was up to. She visited once in three years. I used to write to her often, begging her to come home, but she would not reply to my letters. Oh, how I longed to see her. She broke my heart.

Jo met some friend who said he could get him a job but it was in Yorkshire; I thought it was important for him to go. He left school, went north and got some job at the Cooperative shop. He came home every Easter and Christmas and brought us presents. Tom missed him badly.

Tom received a letter to say he had to go to a special school in Sevenoaks and would live in, coming home at weekends, I visited the school and it seems OK. It was an all-boys' school.

Another chapter in my life was ending for me. Babs gone, Jo and now Tom. I was so unhappy with life. The only good thing ever to happen to me was getting a career, but I would not lose heart. I was on my own all week. I attended flowering-arranging when I was off-duty, and pursued a theory course with the Institute of Domestic Arts on cake icing. This kept my mind occupied. I gave Tom a lot of my time when he came home, and then I took him back on Sunday afternoons for school on Mondays. He was very reluctant to go back until he got used to the idea that he had to be away. He took part in woodwork and swimming; he won a few prizes and made me a wooden box and a cross. I was pleased with his progress, but he often ran away with a friend.

*

Love is in the air. While I was visiting a patient of mine, some of her family was there and I was introduced to them. One in particular was a tall, redheaded, handsome man, who looked very charming.

I was about to leave when he came and took my bags, helped me into my car, shook my hand and said goodbye. Well, I was flattered; I thought he was a nice fellow and wouldn't mind meeting him again; after all I was now

The Tale of a Widow's Anguish

forty and if someone came along, who was sincere, kind and loving, I would certainly get married. I went along to my work and went home, but couldn't help thinking he was indeed a charmer. I slept well that night.

I had completed my care for this patient and she gave me a present; some did in those days. I was delighted; a box of chocolates. She gave me a note as well and said it was a contact number for her brother. He had asked her to give it to me, and asked if I would give her my address and telephone number to pass on to him. I had mixed feelings, but wrote it out and gave it to her.

During that week, I received a phone call. He said it was Dave, whom I had met at his sister's house. He asked how I was and would like to go for a drink one evening? I said I would think about it. He was polite and said he would call again by the end of that week. I had to go for Tom, but I did not mention anything about Dave in case he was not able to take to such matters. In the middle of the week, Dave called to ask if he could meet me at a pub or restaurant. I said yes, as long as it was before Friday. I did not say why; if he asked, then I would explained the situation.

*

We met at seven o'clock on Thursday evening. He gave me a peck on the cheek and asked what I would like to drink. I said lemonade or Coke, and we found a quiet corner. I sipped my drink slowly. I was very nervous and my knees was shaking. He could not see them because I had them well under the table. He said I looked worried and I should have something stronger. I told him I did not drink alcohol and that I never went into a pub. He said I must have lived a sheltered life. I said he could call it that if he liked. He asked if I was ready to eat. I said I was not hungry, but if he wanted to eat I would have something very light.

We chatted over our meal and he asked about my work. I told him it was very rewarding and I was enjoying every minute of it. I asked if he was married. He told me he was separated and lived in digs, as he had been thrown out of his home by his wife. He had two children – a boy and a girl. I asked what he was going to do. He replied that he was looking for a nice lady like me. I asked how he would get home, and I offered him a lift. We did not say too much as I had to concentrate on my driving; a left and right and we were there. We said our goodbyes and I drove home.

We became good friends and he was someone I thought about. We met up regularly and when Tom met him, they struck up a friendship straight away. The three of us went to Yorkshire to see Jo and he was also pleased to meet Dave. Two years' later we got engaged, after his divorce came through. We set a date for the wedding and told the boys, who were happy for us. Babs was contacted, but still kept away. We got married at a registry office, with just the two witnesses and some well-wishers.

Dave moved in to my house. I told him I would like to keep my independence, if he did not mind. He reassured me he would try to be a good husband; if we disagreed about anything, he said, we must talk it over at once. I agreed that that was a good idea. Here was a man who understood about family life. But then I asked him what went wrong to bring about his divorce. He said that his ex told him she was pregnant and in those days parents were strict, and so he had married her. But there was no love because when they did get married, she was not pregnant. But because he was a Christian, he did not want to leave her. Later they did have two children. I did not want to hear any more. I told him we would try and be good to each other.

He was a good father to his children and met up with them often and took Tom out, he taught him how to travel on the trains and buses. Dave was very helpful, loving and kind; he would give his last penny to me. My family back home was pleased for me, especially Ree and Dad. For the rest of my family, I was dead; because he was English they did not want to know. Well, I was happy and had someone to lean on if there was a crisis.

At the end of the month, Tom left school; he was now eighteen years old. It was time for us to help him get a job. Dave knew some people who worked at a nearby bakery, and asked one of them if they were taking apprentices. Dave was told that Tom must go to the bakery on Monday morning. Tom went and got the job; in those days it was 'who you know'.

Tom was excited and went to the bakery each day. Some days he came home with flour all over his head and overalls. He would help to rinse it out, and was pleased with himself. Jo came as usual for the holidays. He had changed jobs many times. I would send him money to help buy clothes, but on the whole he was managing well. Tom was pleased to see him when he came home. Dave and I talked about getting a bigger place; another room would come in handy. We decided to start house-hunting.

A message arrived to say my dad was very ill and wanted to see me, but I couldn't just down tools and go. I discussed the situation with Dave, who said I must ask for some time off. Next day, I contacted County Hall and asked to speak to our manager. She was nice and said I must discuss the situation with my colleagues. I rang around and met up with them the following day, they all agreed to cover for me so I could have two weeks off. I was thankful and went home and told Dave and we both went to the travel agent's to book my return trip.

Tom was told that I would be away for two weeks and Dave would look after him; they would be company for each other. Jo said he would be over at the weekend. We couldn't contact Babs as she kept away from us and had never come home in the last five years. I would often go in search for her; our meeting place was in a restaurant and I would always treat her; never once did she offer to pay for a coffee.

The time came, and Dave and Tom saw me off at the airport. I reached home safely. I felt great; at last I wouldn't have to look over my shoulder to see if any of my enemies were around. Ree and one of her sons came to the airport to meet me. She said Dad had had a stroke but it was too early to say how badly his speech was affected. I went to the hospital. He knew it was me. I squeezed his hand and gave him a hug; he responded with a sheepish smile. We went back to Ree's to catch up with the family gossip and for me to fill her in with my new life. My brother-in-law was pleased for me. I showed the photographs of Dave and myself with the boys and they all wished me well for the future, asking whether I would have children. I said no, that I had enough and Dave felt the same as me; we just wanted some happiness.

Dad seemed to make some progress and I had to leave

The Tale of a Widow's Anguish

in a day or two. We met up with one of my aunts while crossing on the ferry. I went over to say hello. She turned her back quickly and moved away.

I was humiliated and did not follow her; she said something to Ree. My sister declined to say anything. I said I would not buy friends or family. We went home, and I packed and got ready to fly home. We left home and I was ready to get on my plane, sad for Dad but glad I had seen him. My sister said that if Dad died, I must not make a return journey as it cost too much and I might not be able to get leave. We shook hands, kisses and hugs, a few tears but they were happy for me, and I was more than pleased to have seen them again.

Arriving in London, Dave was there to meet me with a red rose in his hand, all smiles. I told him he was a lovely and romantic husband. He asked about my dad and the family at home and I filled him in with the details. I then asked about Tom; Dave seemed reluctant to say anything and went quiet. I asked what was wrong.

He replied that Tom must be OK. Immediately, my instinct told me something was wrong. Dave said we should leave the details till we reach home. I went to check Tom's room; all his clothes had gone. I sat down. Dave went and made us a cup of tea. I kept my cool, waiting to hear where Tom was. Jo had come down the weekend I was away, and Tom had told him he wanted to go and live with him as he did not like where we lived. Jo did not want to take him and told Tom to wait until I was back home.

Jo was cross with him and Dave couldn't persuade him to stay. Dave had told him he was doing well and one day he would be a baker. He did not listen; he packed and Dave took them to the station. Dave was very upset because he thought I would blame him for not being kind to Tom while I was away.

I was concerned for Tom as he was so naive and people would take advantage of him. The devil was at large again, so Dave and I drove to Hull and found Tom in a small, cold, dark room with dirty curtains; a run-down place not fit for human habitation. I tried asking him to come back home, but he told me harshly that he was old enough to look after himself. I gave him money to pay his rent, as he had no job. I asked Jo to keep in touch and let me know how Tom was getting on. We drove home. I was very tense and did not like to leave Tom but he knew he could always return home and we would look after him. Dave said he would learn from making mistakes and we could always go and fetch him back.

On my way home, I said life was so unfair; I had just begun to enjoy my new life with a husband whom I had chosen, and now Tom was making me unhappy. We arrived home and settled down for the night. I told Dave not to let these things come between us; it was no fault of his. He accepted this and we had a good night.

Life went on with just the two of us. We missed Tom but kept in touch quite often. Jo found him new digs and I was pleased that he got a part-time job, which helped him financially.

We saw a new bungalow for sale in the papers, and we called the private owner. He said it was for a quick sale, that the property was left by his late aunt to him and his sister, who wished to sell it. We told him of our interest in buying it, but said we had to sell our house first. He gave us his solicitor's telephone number and address to contact him. We called the solicitor, telling him we wished to purchase the property, but we needed to view

The Tale of a Widow's Anguish

it at the weekend. He agreed and said he would send us a map. Dave told him not to as it would take too long to reach us; we would find our way. On the Saturday we set off early with a packed lunch. After much traffic, we found the little village, and there was this new bungalow with overgrown hedges and a garden with three-foot weeds.

We looked around for a while, then the owner came with the keys. He unlocked the door and we went in. It had a nice large sitting room, three bedrooms, adequate space for cupboards, large front and back gardens and a garage; we were very interested. We stopped for lunch, which we ate in the car. Dave said it was a good house but worried about getting a job. I told him he would have to take any job, if he really wanted to move; as for me, there were lots of jobs as they were crying out for midwives. We arrived home and did some serious talking, and made a list for and against. The 'for' outweighed the 'against', so we decided to put our house on the market the next week. It was in the Seventies, and houses were selling. A man came from the estate agent's and gave us the valuation; we agreed and the board went up. The next day, we were called to say two people wanted to view the property.

I was elated and so was Dave. We showed the people around and they were interested. The first lady was from Bolton. She said she would buy our house; she was so sure I never saw a person so confident. Then the next person came and said they would call our agents later. It was about two hours later that we had a call from the agency to say they had received an offer from the first lady who had visited earlier.

★

There would be big changes now. The boys came home and we told them of our move. Jo was pleased. We would be nearer and they could visit more often. I was looking through *Nursing Times* to seek out a job. A friend suggested I write to all the local authorities asking them if they had any vacancies, which I did. Dave would wait until we moved. It took twelve weeks but the move went well. Jo and Tom came to help us, as we moved ourselves. Since it was a new place, there was nothing much to be done, only some dusting, because no one had ever lived in it.

One thing bothered me; it had coal central heating as there was no gas in this village, only electricity. Dave said he would help with the coal fire. Most of our neighbours were farmers or worked on the land. They were friendly and they told us about the coal man and when he came, as well as the cattle and fruit and vegetable market. Often they left us plants and apples outside the front door.

I got a job as a community nurse and, as it was very rural, I had to do lots of driving, I sometimes did 140 miles per day; patients could live ten or fifteen miles apart; only the RAF houses were together. I was really tired when I got home, but Dave was helpful; we made the arrangement that whoever got home first, started the cooking and lit the fire. We had a weekly menu list. I was hopeless at lighting the fire. One afternoon I came in first to try to clean the grate, and lots of the ashes fell on the carpet. I was furious with myself. This is what country life is all about, I consoled myself.

At weekends, Dave would go and see his father and his children and I would go to Hull to see the boys.

Letters and presents were sent to Dad and Ree, as I appreciated their love and kindness to me; I liked to exhibit my love for everyone, because they would not always be there.

*

Tom's behaviour was becoming more complex and difficult and Jo said I had to take him home. He came home but was always fighting and in a blazing mood. In desperation I sought help and saw our GP, who said he would refer Tom to a social worker. Someone saw him; he had behavioural problems. One evening he went mad, shouting crude language. I was frightened; I could see that one remark would kindle an inferno of emotional harm to him. Dave diverted his flame of anger, to keep Tom from striking the matches. I admired him for his tact.

Tom packed, broke a window and ran away. We called the police and they found him at the railway station, with one of the guards. They brought him home. I called the doctor who referred him to a psychiatrist. I took some time off to be with him, to try to talk to him. I sobbed my eyes out. I felt that nothing would ever be right in my life; the little happiness I was enjoying would be gone, and Dave would leave me with all that was happening. He did not; he was very supportive indeed.

Tom saw the specialist, who gave him some pills for his problem. It was working and he responded well, but after three months he stopped taking them, saying he didn't need them. Jo had decided to return home, and had rented a caravan not far from home. He got a job at a poultry factory. He was there a few months and helped

Tom to get a job too. Things were looking good; Jo was happy in his job and so was Tom. Jo bought a new house. I helped with the deposit. It was a three-bedroom house, so Tom went to live with him. They got on well for a short time, but then trouble began. Tom was bad-tempered and hit Jo and hurt him badly. Jo, such a good-natured person, forgave him. Tom had a fight with one of the workers and lost his job. More rebelling now, as he had idle time. He was discharged from the social worker so I took him to work with me some days to lessen his boredom. I gave him magazines and puzzles to do while I went in to see the patients, but I was always so tense when he was with me. He was not the lovable Tom I knew. I told him if he would like to live by himself, I would help him get a small house. He said that would be nice; it was the first time in a while he had shown any interest in what I had to say. I was delighted.

I told Dave of my idea. He asked if we could afford it; I told him we could, so we went flat-hunting for Tom. There were some small houses suitable for Tom; we picked a two-bedroom bungalow which would be ready in a few months. Tom was pleased. I would try to train him how to pay his bills. I drew up a list of all the utilities bills and told him to set aside the money for them. He was receiving benefits at that time, and I planned to give him extra money for food and clothing. He took it all in and seemed pleased, and we began to shop for his new place.

*

I sent a ticket for my sister to come and see us. It was summer and she would be with us for three months; by then, Tom's bungalow would be ready and he would have moved in. We all had a wonderful summer and we took my sister to see some interesting places, which she enjoyed. Her holiday ended and she returned home with some happy memories, which she told the family.

Tom's home was completed and he moved in. Every other day I called in to see him, and we kept an eye on all his bills, getting him to pay them as they came in. We put in all off-peak heaters and he had electricity on a meter, so he would have fewer bills coming in. He managed to get a part-time job as a handyman. Dave said we needed a break and he suggested we visit my sister and Dad as he was back on his feet, and the Tiger had died.

We booked a ticket for two weeks. Jo was asked if he would check up on Tom while we were away. He promised, saying he would stay with him for company until we got back. Plans were made and we reassured Tom that Jo would spend the two weeks with him while we were away.

*

All was set for us to see Dad and the family. We had a warm welcome, Dad was happy for me and some of the family came to see us. Dave enjoyed himself as it was his first visit to South America. They made a lot of fuss and most evenings we ate our meals outside. We both enjoyed ourselves until it was time for us to leave. I was sad to see Dad cry for the first time in my life; everyone shed a few tears. On arriving home I called Tom to see if he was OK, he said that Jo had stayed with him and he did most of the cooking.

More disruption. Tom met a scruffy man who talked

his way into his home and encouraged Tom to play his music very loud. His neighbours complained to me when I visited Tom. I asked Tom if it was true. He said he had the right to have anyone in his home. I told him to let only nice people in, and that he must not play his music to annoy his neighbours. He was rude. I left and went home, but soon received a call from someone who did not want to give their name, but said I had to visit at once or else the police would be called in. Dave was tired and said I should go but if I needed him, to call him on the phone. I got there and all hell broke loose. Tom was shouting at the top of his voice. The scruffy man seemed to need a bath and was smoking.

I told him to leave, as he was not good company for my son, and nobody smokes in our house. I went into the spare bedroom only to find black bags tied up and lots of dirty cups in the room. I ordered him to leave. Tom protested; I told him that I was responsible for the property. He left, swearing and using crude language. Tom went in the kitchen and smashed some glasses, throwing things through the window. I told him to calm down. I saw a brown envelope with a strange name on it; it was a discharge note from a prison. I got goose pimples and was frightened, as I thought this man had just come out of prison and, looking for lodgings, Tom was an easy target to pick on. However, Tom left the house and I was sick with worry as I didn't what was going on in his head. I went home and told Dave about the saga; for the first time, he didn't know what on earth we could do.

My patience was running out; I felt like Job. We asked the church to pray for Tom and us. He was not working again and for him to sign on the DSS meant waiting for several weeks. I paid all the bills and left food for him each day on my way home. I complained to Dave, who said things would change. I wondered whether for better or worse.

Months later, Tom was back on benefits, but this time he would not pay any bills that came in. I told him there were no free lunches and he had to pay up, otherwise they would stop all the services provided for him. He told Jo he was going to get a motorbike and he was saving up for it. I told Jo to tell him it was not a good idea.

Tom bought his motorbike. Not many days after, he came off the bike, broke his arm and was hospitalised for a few weeks. The bike was a write-off and the HP still had to be paid. I was furious; we were going to and from the hospital each day, which meant lots of strain and mental fatigue.

I said to Dave that my life had been spent with grief and sighing; fear was always at the back of my mind. The bike had to be paid off so I went with Tom and settled the bill. He was not covered by the insurance. I told him he had to pay his outgoings, and no more bike. When he was fit, I bought him a pedal bike so he could get around, but a few months later he gave it away. I told him the bike was for him and he must ask the person to return the bike. He was aggressive, saying he would do what he pleased. This time, I would have to go and retrieve the bike. Jo got the address and we went and fetched it and brought it back to our house. Tom went mad and did not want to speak to us. Months went by. I continued to visit his home, leaving money and loving notes. No response. Dave said to leave him. Tom visited Jo but he said little and was very moody.

★

Dave contracted a nasty cold and was unable to shake it off. He saw the doctor, who told him he would like him to have an X-ray. Dave went, and two weeks later he was asked to see the doctor again, who said he wanted him to have a scan. He was getting breathless, and all the remedies given did not help. Dave took it lightly and said it would go when it was ready; I was concerned. He told me not to worry as I had enough to cope with: Tom was still at loggerheads with me. I had retired now, so Dave and I spent more time together. I had signed up for some voluntary work – Home Start.

The nightmare began. Dave went for a scan. When the doctor saw the results he asked Dave if he could see a dark area all around the ribcage. Dave said he didn't know what it all meant. The man was tactless and told him he had cancer; the dreaded thing no one wants to hear. The morning before he went for the scan, I had told him I could go with him; he said no. When Dave came home, a few minutes passed until I was back from the charity work. I shouted, as usual, that I was home, but there was no reply. Dave was sitting in the sitting room crying his head off. He asked why I took so long to come home. I sat on the arm of the chair and gave him a big hug, asking him what was wrong. He sobbed more and I too started crying. He told me he would be leaving me soon. I told him not to be so daft.

He said he had cancer of both lungs and the kidneys. I asked how could this be; I did not know what to say to him – I was lost for words – such a turning point in our life. Oh, how I cried in the kitchen; I was numb. I called Jo and he came and offered to make us a light supper but our appetite had gone. Dave was silent and we put him to bed. He was shivering and his face was very pale.

The Tale of a Widow's Anguish

I called our doctor out and told him about the scan. He said the result should have gone to him first and he would have broken the news. The doctor gave Dave some Valium to sleep and said there was lots of treatment available and Dave must not worry, as it may not be as bad as the man had told him. We thought there was hope and Dave calmed down.

We managed to get some sleep and Dave had a little to eat. He rang our solicitor to say he wanted to make a will. He was told to call in the next day. I went with him but left to do some shopping. We both went to the bank where he withdrew some money and said we should go to a jeweller's. He said to the salesperson that he would like to buy his wife a Gucci watch! Despite my protests, he insisted, saying it was my last birthday present and I must have it. I had to leave the shop for a moment, crying my eyes out. The lady came out and told me to come in and see which one I would like. Reluctantly, I picked one. Dave was pleased, and paid for it. We went home; he was so breathless, I had a job to get him to bed.

Late that night, I had to call the doctor out. The GP came and sent Dave to the hospital. He went to casualty and was transferred to a ward where he saw the consultant and had his lungs drained. The next day he could breathe quite normally, but the doctors said he had to stay in for another few days. Later that week, he was discharged.

The GP put him on morphine sulphate to kill the pain, and Valium three times a day. This helped him cope, but he was losing his mind. His lungs filled up again and he was unable to breathe; it was in and out of hospital. I was looking after him single-handed, until one day, I had a visit from a nurse from the local hospice, who said they would come in for a few hours, so I could go shopping. It was really hard work caring for him, as he was unable to walk now and had to use a wheelchair. He was now incontinent and his body was not functioning any more.

His request was that he wanted to die at home, but I was cracking up. The last time he went into the hospital, he fell out of bed and sustained terrible head injuries. I was called to go and see him. He was semi-conscious when I got there and his forehead was swollen with mighty bruising. I was talking to him to wake him up. The consultant came to see him and asked me whether he was responding to my call. I was so angry. I said Dave was not only dying of cancer but would die of head injuries.

The hospice doctor came and saw Dave and gave him forty-eight hours. I was told to prepare myself for the worst. I moved into the ward to care for him. All fluid and medication was stopped.

Two days later, while I was giving him a wash, Dave said with a forceful voice that he was hungry. Surprised indeed, I gave him some water, and rushed to make him some porridge with lots of milk. I fed him and he ate the lot and wanted a second helping. He was fully conscious. I was so happy; I thought he was responding to treatment and might perhaps live a few more years, but, as he was weak, the hospital suggested he went into a nursing home. I was given a list to choose one for him. I started ringing round to make appointments to visit some of the homes I thought would be suitable as I wanted the best for him. I found a top-grade one, but I would have to pay the extra money. I visited him and told him it would only be for a short time until he became stronger; he was a bit resentful, but responded to gentle persuasion.

The Tale of a Widow's Anguish

I went and saw my ninety-four-year-old lady and her son to tell them my news. When I got there, Tom was there. He began saying I was a no-good mum. I said I did not come here to speak to you. He came over to where I sat and put his large hands around my neck, choking me, causing constriction in my neck. I was unable to breathe, the dear old lady was shouting that he was going to kill me and to stop. Her son did not say anything. I was terrified; I thought he would strangle me to death as I was helpless. The lady's son was frightened as well. I wanted to call the police but thought they would put him away. I came home lonely and empty inside, crying my eyes out, failing to understand why I had to endure such misery year after year. The ordeal seemed endless. I called Social Services, who weren't much help. The lady said to call the police the next time he attacked me. I thought there might not be another time; given a chance, he would kill me. I went to bed with nobody to talk to. This is when I missed Dave the most; he was my backup and a shoulder to cry on, and I couldn't tell him.

Dave was now in the nursing home. I went and saw him. He said he went outside looking for me and fell over. The nurse had to fetch him in. I told him if he wanted to go out, I could push him in the wheelchair. He agreed, so the next day I took him out. He looked around, and he said he would like to come out again. I told him we would. He was going downhill fast and he said he would not be here next week. My heart was weeping inside but I hid the tears. I said to tell me anything; he said he wanted to cry but was unable to. I think it was the drugs he was on. I usually stayed until he was ready for bed then I would dress him and settle him in. I would say a little prayer before leaving and then walk home sadly.

★

Tom was behaving badly, fighting with his neighbours and writing abusive letters to them. He made a lot of enemies and they came to my house and complained about him many times. The police were called out and sometimes I had the police knocking at my door. How I wished I was the one dying and not Dave! People like Tom do not admit that they have a problem and will not go for treatment; he lacked understanding and reasoning. How I wished for a human heart to listen to me.

Next day, a call came from Matron to say Dave wanted me to come and sit with him. It was early morning but I got over there as quick as I could. He seemed bright and wanted his nails and hair cut, so this was done. Then he said he fancied cherry brandy. I said that was a tall order, but I went and told Matron of his request. She said to go and get him a bottle. I asked what about the medication he was taking, but she said when one is dying, little harm can be done. I looked in my purse and I only had £10. I hoped it would be enough to get a bottle. I went into shops, pubs, everywhere and finally found the only one in a wine shop; it cost £9.99. I went back and asked again how much he could have. As much as he wanted, was the answer – I gave him a snap glass full. He drank it and said I must have the rest; I took a little sip, to please him really. This was our farewell parting. I spent the night with him; he was on his way. It was an agonising night. I came home and asked the priest to go and see him. Then I hurried back, only to see the priest waiting at the door for me. I knew he was gone.

I screamed my head off, saying I had told him to wait, I would be back. But time and tide wait for no man. I was numb with sadness, but his suffering was ended. This was a crucial time; all arrangements had to be made quickly. I only had two days. The priest was good. We talked about Dave's request, as he wanted to be buried quickly, and have only the family present. I tried to fulfil all his requests.

It was the longest and saddest night I spent all alone in my house. Tom was not living far away, but he did not come or want to know; Babs and Jo rang but that was all. When I think about the millions of people out there, even the so-called Christians did not offer to come and sit with me; my world had crumbled.

Distressed and distraught, nevertheless I had to keep going. Sometimes I fail to understand why I should have such a burden. I have asked for help for Tom but the answer is always he – Tom – has to ask for help. The law really needs to be changed; only when Tom kills me, God forbid, will he get help. In the meantime, mental and physical exhaustion will take me, hopefully, to my grave. I am not morbid; this is just the reality of my life. How I long to have a quiet life. Only God knows, but my times are in his hands; he knows the number of my days.

Those of you out there, I hope you have better days than I had. This is the true story of my life. I wish it was better. I live in hope, and wait for God's calling.

*With Compliment
Abiwata
Manrou*

Printed in the United Kingdom
by Lightning Source UK Ltd.
108869UKS00002B/403-423